Virtual Medical Offi

for

Young: Kinn's The Administrative Medical Assistant,
7th Edition

Virtual Medical Office

for

Young: Kinn's The Administrative Medical Assistant, 7th Edition

Study Guide prepared by

Tracie Fuqua, B.S., CMA(AAMA)

Program Director
Medical Assistant Program
Wallace State Community College
Hanceville, Alabama

Textbook by

Alexandra Patricia Young-Adams, BBA, RMA, CMA(AAMA)

Adjunct Instructor
Everest College, Arlington Midcities Campus
Arlington, Texas
Professional Writer
Grand Prairie, Texas

Formerly
Director of Admissions
Parker College of Chiropractic
Dallas, Texas

Formerly
Program Director
Medical/Assisting/HIM Programs
Ultrasound Diagnostic School
Irving, Texas

software developed by

Wolfsong Informatics, LLC
Tucson, Arizona

SAUNDERS

ELSEVIER

SAUNDERS
ELSEVIER

3251 Riverport Lane
Maryland Heights, Missouri 63043

VIRTUAL MEDICAL OFFICE FOR
YOUNG: KINN'S THE ADMINISTRATIVE MEDICAL ASSISTANT
SEVENTH EDITION
Copyright © 2011, 2007 by Saunders, an imprint of Elsevier Inc.

ISBN: 978-1-4377-2402-8

Notice

Knowledge and best practice in this field are constantly changing. As new research and experience broaden our knowledge, changes in practice, treatment and drug therapy may become necessary or appropriate. Readers are advised to check the most current information provided (i) on procedures featured or (ii) by the manufacturer of each product to be administered, to verify the recommended dose or formula, the method and duration of administration, and contraindications. It is the responsibility of the practitioner, relying on their own experience and knowledge of the patient, to make diagnoses, to determine dosages and the best treatment for each individual patient, and to take all appropriate safety precautions. To the fullest extent of the law, neither the Publisher nor the Authors assumes any liability for any injury and/or damage to persons or property arising out or related to any use of the material contained in this book.

ISBN: 978-1-4377-2402-8

Acquisitions Editor: Susan Cole
Developmental Editor: Karen Baer
Publishing Services Manager: Gayle May
Project Manager: Stephen Bancroft

Printed in the United States of America

Last digit is the print number: 9 8 7 6 5 4 3 2

Table of Contents

Getting Started

■ LOGIN AND ENROLLMENT INSTRUCTIONS

Please check with your instructor prior to registering to verify whether you are required to enroll in the instructor's *Virtual Medical Office* course on Evolve. If so, your instructor will provide you with your course ID and you will use the steps under **Instructor-Led Course** on the following page.

SELF-STUDY COURSE

1. To access your Virtual Medical Office, please visit http://evolve.elsevier.com/Kinn/admin.
2. Select the **Simulations—VMO** tab and click **Register for These Simulations** to begin the one-time-only registration process.
3. Select **I already have an Access code** and enter the code located on the inside front cover of this study guide exactly as it appears.
4. Click **Register**.
5. If you already have an Evolve account or have previously requested products from Evolve, provide your case-sensitive username and password in the Returning User area and click **Login**. If you do not have an Evolve account, provide your desired password for the account in the New User area and click **Continue**. Provide the required profile information and click **Continue**.
6. Read the Registered User Agreement. Check **Yes, I accept this agreement** and then click **Submit**.
7. A screen confirming your enrollment will appear. Click **My Home**.
8. This product will be added to your Evolve account under the My Content area located on the left-hand side of the Evolve homepage. Click to expand the **Simulations—VMO** heading and then click the link titled **Young: Kinn's The Administrative Assistant, Seventh Edition**.
9. Click **Simulations—VMO** to access your activities.
10. Your case-sensitive account information will be emailed to you. Please note your account information. If needed, you can request your account information at any time by clicking on the **I forgot my login information** link on the Evolve homepage.
11. Please bookmark this page (http://evolve.elsevier.com/student) to easily log in and access your *Virtual Medical Office* in the future.

INSTRUCTOR-LED COURSE

1. Go to http://evolve.elsevier.com/enroll.

2. Enter the **Course ID** provided to you by your instructor and click the arrow button.

3. Verify that the course information is correct and check **Yes, this is my course**.

4. Select **I already have an Access code** and enter the code located on the inside front cover of this study guide exactly as it appears.

5. Click **Register**.

6. If you already have an Evolve account or have previously requested products from Evolve, provide your case-sensitive username and password in the Returning User area and click **Login**. If you do not have an Evolve account, provide your desired password for the account in the New User area and click **Continue**. Provide the required profile information and click **Continue**.

7. Read the Registered User Agreement. Check **Yes, I accept this agreement** and click **Submit**.

8. A screen confirming your enrollment will appear. Click **Get Started** or **My Home**.

9. This product will be added to your Evolve account under the My Content area located on the left-hand side of the Evolve homepage. Click to expand the **Simulations—VMO** heading and then click **Young: Kinn's The Administrative Assistant, Seventh Edition**.

10. Click **Course Documents** and then click **Simulations—VMO** to access your activities.

11. Your case-sensitive account information will be emailed to you. Please note your account information. If needed, you can request your account information at any time by clicking on **I forgot my login information** on the Evolve homepage.

12. Please bookmark this page (http://evolve.elsevier.com/student) to easily log in and access your *Virtual Medical Office* in the future.

■ **SUPPORT INFORMATION**

Visit the Evolve Support Portal at http://evolvesupport.elsevier.com to access the Evolve Knowledge Base, Downloads, Hours of Operation, and Support Ticket System. Live Evolve Support is available by calling 1-800-222-9570.

GETTING SET UP

■ TECHNICAL REQUIREMENTS

To use an Evolve Online Product, you will need access to a computer that is connected to the Internet and equipped with web browser software that supports frames. For optimal performance, it is recommended that you have speakers and use a high-speed Internet connection. Dial-up modems are not recommended for *Virtual Medical Office*.

WINDOWS®

Windows PC
Windows XP, Windows Vista™
Pentium® processor (or equivalent) @ 1 GHz (Recommend 2 GHz or better)
800 x 600 screen size
Thousands of colors
Soundblaster 16 soundcard compatibility
Stereo speakers or headphones
Internet Explorer (IE) version 6.0 or higher
Mozilla Firefox version 2.0 or higher

MACINTOSH®

Mozilla Firefox version 2.0 or higher

■ WEB BROWSERS

Supported web browsers include Microsoft Internet Explorer (IE) version 7.0 or higher and Mozilla Firefox version 3.0 or higher.

If you use America Online® (AOL) for web access, you will need AOL version 4.0 or higher, and one of the browsers listed above. Earlier versions of AOL and Internet Explorer will not run the course properly and you will have difficulty accessing many features.

For best results with AOL:
- Connect to the Internet using AOL version 4.0 or higher.
- Open a private chat within AOL. (This allows the AOL client to remain open, without asking if you wish to disconnect while minimized.)
- Minimize AOL.
- Launch one of the recommended browsers.

■ **SCREEN SETTINGS**

For best results, your computer monitor resolution should be set at a minimum of 800 x 600. The number of colors displayed should be set to "thousands or higher" (High Color or 16 bit) or "millions of colors" (True Color or 24 bit).

WINDOWS

1. From the **Start** menu, select **Settings**, then **Control Panel**.
2. Double-click on the **Display** icon.
3. Click on the **Settings** tab.
4. Under **Screen resolution** use the slider bar to select **800 x 600 pixels**.
5. Access the **Colors** drop-down menu by clicking on the down arrow.
6. Select **High Color (16 bit)** or **True Color (24 bit)**.
7. Click on **Apply**, then **OK**.
8. You may be asked to verify the setting changes. Click **Yes**.
9. You may be asked to restart your computer to accept the changes. Click **Yes**.

MACINTOSH

1. Select the **Monitors** control panel.
2. Select **800 x 600** (or greater) from the **Resolution** area.
3. Select **Thousands** or **Millions** from the **Color Depth** area.

Enable Cookies

Browser	Steps
Internet Explorer (IE) 7.0 or higher	1. Select **Tools → Internet Options**. 2. Select **Privacy** tab. 3. Click the **Advanced** button. 4. Click the check box next to **Override Automatic Cookie Handling**. 5. Click the **Accept** radio buttons under **First-party Cookies** and **Third-party Cookies**. 6. Click the box for **Always allow session cookies**. 7. Click **OK**. 8. Click **OK**.
Mozilla Firefox 3.0 or higher	1. Select **Tools → Options**. 2. Select the **Privacy** tab. 3. Assure that **Use custom settings for history** is selected in the drop-down menu. 4. Check the box for **Accept Cookies from Sites**. 5. Check the box for **Accept third-party cookies**. 6. Click **OK**.

Set Cache to Always Reload a Page

Browser	Steps
Internet Explorer (IE) 7.0 or higher	1. Select **Tools → Internet Options**. 2. Select **General** tab. 3. Click the button for **Settings** in the Browsing History Section. 4. Click the radio button for **Every time I visit the webpage**. 5. Enter in **0** (or smallest number allowed) in the Disk space to Use section. 6. Click **OK**. 7. Click **OK**.
Mozilla Firefox 3.0 or higher	1. Select **Tools → Options**. 2. Select the **Privacy** icon. 3. Click to expand Cache. 4. Set the value to "0" in the **Use up to: __ MB of disk space for the cache** field. 5. Click **OK**.

Plug-Ins

 Adobe Acrobat Reader—With the free Acrobat Reader software, you can view and print Adobe PDF files. Many Evolve products offer student and instructor manuals, checklists, and more in this format!

Download at: http://www.adobe.com

 Apple QuickTime—Install this to hear word pronunciations, heart and lung sounds, and many other helpful audio clips within Evolve Online Courses!

Download at: http://www.apple.com

 Adobe Flash Player—This player will enhance your viewing of many Evolve web pages, as well as educational short-form to long-form animation within the Evolve Learning System!

Download at: http://www.adobe.com

 Adobe Shockwave Player—Shockwave is best for viewing the many interactive learning activities within Evolve Online Courses!

Download at: http://www.adobe.com

 Microsoft Word Viewer—With this viewer Microsoft Word users can share documents with those who don't have Word, and users without Word can open and view Word documents. Many Evolve products have testbank, student and instructor manuals, and other documents available for downloading and viewing on your own computer!

Download at: http://www.microsoft.com

Office Tour

Welcome to *Virtual Medical Office*, a virtual office setting in which you can work with multiple patient simulations and also learn to access and evaluate the information resources that are essential for providing high-quality medical assistance.

In the virtual medical office, Mountain View Clinic, you can access the Reception area, Exam Room, Laboratory, Office Manager, and Check Out area, plus a separate room for Billing and Coding.

■ BEFORE YOU START

Make sure you have your textbook nearby when you use *Virtual Medical Office* online. You will want to consult topic areas in your textbook frequently while working online and using this study guide.

■ HOW TO SIGN IN

- After entering the access code included inside this study guide, enter your name on the Medical Assistant identification badge.
- Click on **Start Simulation**.

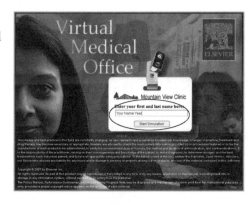

- This takes you to the office map screen. Across the top of this screen is the list of patients available for you to follow throughout their office visit.

■ PATIENT LIST

1. **Janet Jones (age 50)**—Ms. Jones has sustained an on-the-job injury. She is in pain and impatient. By working with Ms. Jones, students will learn about managing difficult patients, as well as the requirements involved in Workers' Compensation cases.

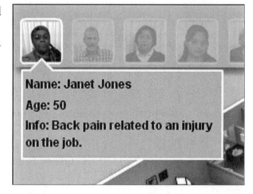

Name: Janet Jones
Age: 50
Info: Back pain related to an injury on the job.

2. **Wilson Metcalf (age 65)**—A Medicare patient, Mr. Metcalf is being seen for multiple symptoms of abdominal pain, nausea, vomiting, and fever. He is seriously ill and might need more specialized care in a hospital setting.

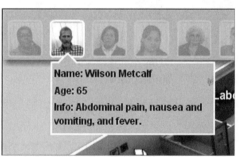

Name: Wilson Metcalf
Age: 65
Info: Abdominal pain, nausea and vomiting, and fever.

3. **Rhea Davison (age 53)**—An established patient with chronic and multiple symptoms, Ms. Davison does not have medical insurance.

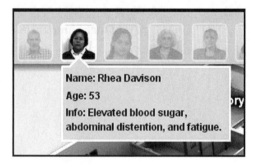

Name: Rhea Davison
Age: 53
Info: Elevated blood sugar, abdominal distention, and fatigue.

4. **Shaunti Begay (age 15)**—A new patient, Shaunti Begay is a minor who has an appointment for a sports physical. Upon arrival, Shaunti and her family learn that Mountain View Clinic does not participate in their health insurance.

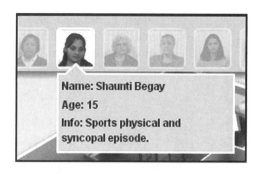

Name: Shaunti Begay
Age: 15
Info: Sports physical and syncopal episode.

5. **Jean Deere (age 83)**—Accompanied by her son, Ms. Deere is an established Medicare patient being evaluated for memory loss and hearing loss.

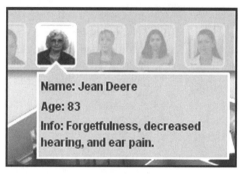

Name: Jean Deere
Age: 83
Info: Forgetfulness, decreased hearing, and ear pain.

6. **Renee Anderson (age 43)**—Ms. Anderson scheduled her appointment for a routine gynecological exam but exhibits symptoms that suggest she is a victim of domestic violence.

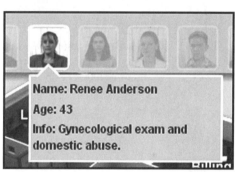

Name: Renee Anderson
Age: 43
Info: Gynecological exam and domestic abuse.

7. **Teresa Hernandez (age 16)**—Teresa is a minor patient who is unaccompanied by a parent for her appointment. She is seeking contraceptive counseling and STD testing.

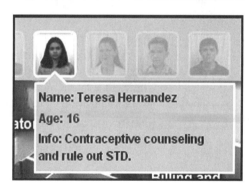

Name: Teresa Hernandez
Age: 16
Info: Contraceptive counseling and rule out STD.

8. **Louise Parlet (age 24)**—Ms. Parlet is an established patient being seen for a pregnancy test and examination. She will also need to be referred to an OB/GYN specialist.

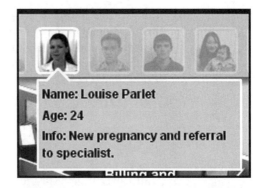

9. **Tristan Tsosie (age 8)**—A minor patient accompanied by his older sister and younger brother, Tristan is having a splint and sutures removed from his injured right arm.

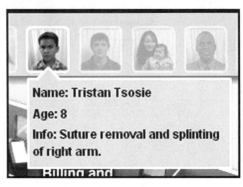

10. **Jose Imero (age 16)**—Jose is a minor patient who is scheduled for an emergency appointment to have the laceration on his foot sutured.

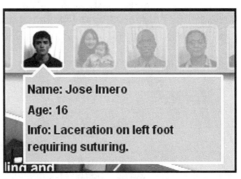

11. **Jade Wong (age 7 months)**—Jade and her parents are new patients to Mountain View Clinic. Jade needs a checkup and updates to her immunizations. Her mother does not speak English.

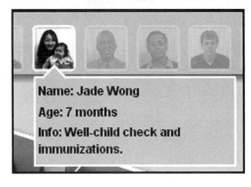

12. **John R. Simmons (age 43)**—Dr. Simmons is a new patient with a history of high blood pressure and recent episodes of blood in his urine.

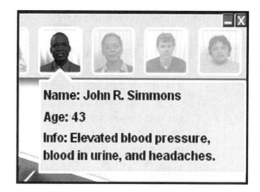

13. **Hu Huang (age 67)**—Mr. Huang developed a severe cough and fever after returning from a recent trip to Asia.

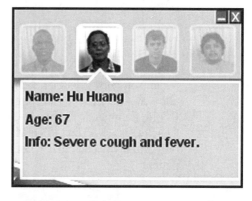

14. **Kevin McKinzie (age 18)**—Mr. McKinzie has made an appointment because of his nausea and vomiting. He is insured through the restaurant where he works.

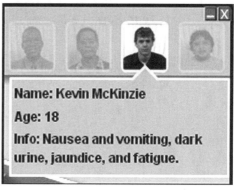

15. **Jesus Santo (age 32)**—Mr. Santo has been brought to the office as a walk-in appointment by his employer for leg pain and a fever. He has no insurance or identification, but his employer has offered to pay for the visit.

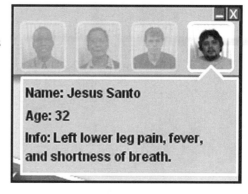

■ BASIC NAVIGATION

HOW TO SELECT A PATIENT

The list of patients is located across the top of the office map screen. Pointing your cursor at the various patients will highlight their photo and reveal their name, age, and medical problem (see examples in the photos on the previous pages). When you click on the patient you wish to review, a larger photo and description will appear in the lower left corner of the screen.

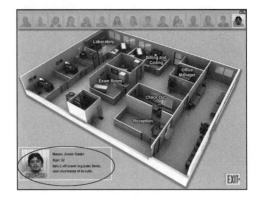

Note: You **must** select a patient before you are allowed access to the Reception area, Exam Room, Laboratory, Billing and Coding office, or Check Out area. The Office Manager area is the only room you can enter without first selecting a patient.

HOW TO SELECT A ROOM

After selecting a patient, use your cursor to highlight the room you want to enter. The active room will be shaded blue on the map. Click to enter the room.

HOW TO LEAVE A ROOM

When you are finished working in a room, you can leave by clicking the exit arrow found at the bottom right corner of the screen.

Leaving a room will automatically take you to the
Summary Menu.

From the Summary Menu, you can choose to:

- **Look at Your Performance Summary**

  In each room there are interactive wizards or tasks that can be completed. The Performance
  Summary lets you compare your answers with those of the experts.

- **Continue with Current Room**

  This takes you back to the last room in which you worked. This option is not available if you
  have already reviewed your Performance Summary.

- **Return to Map**

  This reopens the office map for you to select another room and/or another patient.

- **View Credits for This Program**

  This provides a complete listing of software developers, publisher, and authors.

- **Exit the Program**

  This closes the *Virtual Medical Office* software. You will need to sign in again before you can
  use the program.

HOW TO USE THE PERFORMANCE SUMMARY

If you completed any of the interactive wizards in a room, you can compare your answers with
those of the experts by accessing your Performance Summary. The Performance Summary is not
a grading tool, although it is valuable for self-assessment and review.

From the Summary Menu, click on **Look at Your
Performance Summary**.

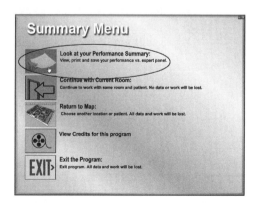

The complete list of tasks associated with the active room will appear with two columns showing the results of your choices. Your answers will appear in the column labeled **Your Performance**, and the answers chosen by the expert will appear in the **Expert's Performance** column. A check mark in the same box in both columns indicates that your answer matched the expert's answer. The Performance Summary can be saved to your computer or disk by clicking on the disk icon at the upper right side of the screen. The saved file can be printed or emailed to your instructor. A hard copy can also be printed without saving by clicking on the printer icon at the upper right corner of the screen.

■ ROOM DESCRIPTIONS

Each room can be entered at any time in any order. You can follow a patient's visit from Reception to Check Out, or you can choose to observe each patient at any point in their care. Below is a description of the information and activities that can be found in various rooms.

ALL ROOMS

- In all rooms you can access the patient's medical record and the office Policy Manual.
- In all rooms in which there are interactive tasks to be completed, you can select tasks or features from the menu on the left of the screen, as shown on this sample of the menu in the Reception area.

- As an alternative to using the menu, you can click on the corresponding items in the photo of the room. As you move your cursor over each item connected to one of the tasks on the menu, it will highlight and become active.

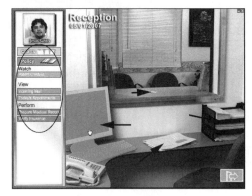

RECEPTION

In the Reception area, you can choose:

- **Charts**—Look at the patient's chart. *Note:* For new patients, there will be no information available in the chart at this time, although you do have the option of assembling a new medical record.
- **Policy**—Open the office Policy Manual and review the established administrative, clinical, and laboratory policies for Mountain View Clinic. Within the Policy Manual you will also find the Coding and Billing Manual.
- **Watch**—Watch a video of the patient's arrival. Each patient is shown checking in at the front desk so that you can observe the procedures typically performed by the receptionist and consider some of the various problems that might arise.
- **Incoming Mail**—Look at the incoming mail for the day. Mountain View Clinic has received a wide range of correspondence that must be read and responded to accordingly.
- **Today's Appointments**—Review the appointment schedule for the day. You can check the schedule to find out what time patients are supposed to arrive, the reason for their visit, and how much time the physician will need for the examination.
- **Prepare Medical Record**—Practice preparing the medical record. This interactive feature allows you to build a medical record for a new patient or update information for an established patient.
- **Verify Insurance**—Verify a patient's insurance. Also interactive, this feature allows you to ask patients about the status of their insurance and to view their insurance cards.

EXAM ROOM

- **Charts** and **Policy**—Access the patient's chart and the office Policy Manual.
- **Watch**—View video clips of different parts of the patient's exam. Observe the actions of the medical assistants in the videos and critique the competencies demonstrated.
- **Exam Notes**—Review the physician's documented findings for the current visit. These notes are added to the full Progress Notes in the patient's chart as the patient continues on to Check Out.
- **Perform**—Perform multiple tasks that are required of a clinical medical assistant, such as preparing the room for the exam, taking vital signs and patient history, and properly positioning the patient for an exam.

LABORATORY

- **Charts** and **Policy**—Access the patient's chart and the office Policy Manual.
- **View: Logs**—View the laboratory's log of specimens sent out for testing. Opportunities to practice filling out laboratory logs are included in the workbook exercises.
- **Perform**—Perform specific tasks as needed in the laboratory, such as collecting and testing specimens. These interactive wizards walk you through the steps for collecting and testing specimens ordered by the physician as part of the patient's examination. The Progress Notes are available throughout so that you can review the physician's directions.

CHECK OUT

- **Charts** and **Policy**—Access the patient's chart and the office Policy Manual.
- **Watch**—Watch a video clip of the patient checking out of the office at the end of the visit. Observe the administrative medical assistants as they schedule follow-up appointments, accept payments, and manage the various duties and problems that may arise.
- **View**—Look at the Encounter Form completed for each patient and verify that the form is filled out correctly and completely.
- **Perform**—Certain patients will require a return visit to the office. Schedule their follow-up appointments as needed. Opportunities to work with the appointment book and additional scheduling tasks are included in the study guide.

BILLING AND CODING

- **View: Aging Report**—Review the outstanding balances on various patient accounts and assess when to implement different collection techniques.
- **View: Encounter Form**—Review the patient's Encounter Form and determine whether the proper procedures were followed to ensure accurate billing and coding.
- **View: Fee Schedule**—Review the office's fee schedule to calculate the proper charges for the patient's visit.

OFFICE MANAGER

- **Policy**—View the office Policy Manual. Note that patient charts are not available from the manager's office, and there is no need to select a patient to enter the Office Manager area.
- **View**—A variety of financial and administrative documents are available for viewing in the manager's office. Banking deposits and payments can be tracked through these documents, and opportunities to practice managing office finances are included in the study guide.
- **Perform: Transcribe Report**—A recorded medical report is included for transcription practice with full player controls.

■ EMBEDDED ERRORS

The individual lessons and patient scenarios associated with the *Virtual Medical Office* program were designed to stimulate critical thinking and analytical skills and to help develop the competencies you will be tested on as part of your course work. Thus deliberate errors have been embedded into each of the 15 patient scenarios and in the Billing and Coding and Office Manager activities. Many of the exercises in the study guide draw attention to these errors so that you can work through how and why a correction needs to be made. Other errors have not been specifically addressed, and you may discover them as you work through the various rooms and tasks. Instructors and students alike are encouraged to use any errors they find to further develop the essential critical thinking and decision-making skills needed for the clinical office.

The following icons are used throughout the study guide to help you quickly identify particular activities and assignments:

 Reading Assignment—tells you which textbook chapter(s) you should read before starting each lesson

 Writing Activity—certain activities focus on written responses such as filling out forms or completing documentation

 Online Activity—marks the beginning of an activity that uses the *Virtual Medical Office* simulation software

 Online Instructions—indicates the steps to follow as you navigate through the software

 Reference—indicates questions and activities that require you to consult your textbook

 Time—indicates the approximate amount of time needed to complete the exercise

LESSON 1

Performing Other Professional Duties

Reading Assignment: Chapter 3—The Medical Assisting Profession
Chapter 4—Professional Behavior in the Workplace
Chapter 5—Interpersonal Skills and Human Behavior

Patient: Rhea Davison

Note: The first exercise does not involve Rhea Davison, but you have to choose a patient to access the clinic rooms.

Learning Objectives:

- Prepare the documentation for possible termination of the patient.
- Describe the necessary documentation of licensure and accreditation.
- Recognize the need for confidentiality and HIPAA regulations.
- Prepare a travel itinerary for a physician who will be speaking at the national AAMA conference.
- Locate resources and information for the employer.
- Describe the need for and the maintenance of liability coverage.

Overview:

In this lesson you will prepare documentation needed for assisting the physician in various areas related to office policies and the physician's professional needs. The ethical and legal aspects of confidentiality are addressed, as well as how to deal with patients who habitually cancel appointments. The Internet will be used to research travel arrangements for a conference one of the physicians needs to attend. Finally, the importance of maintaining liability insurance will be discussed.

Exercise 1

Online Activity—Recognizing the Need for Patient Termination

45 minutes

- Sign in to Mountain View Clinic.
- Select **Rhea Davison** from the patient list and click on **Reception** to be able to access the schedule.

- At the Reception desk, click on **Today's Appointments** to review the day's schedule. You will need to scroll down the appointment book with your mouse to see both the morning and afternoon schedules.

1. Who is the patient who has canceled an appointment, and what was the patient's chief complaint?

Look at your office Policy Manual regarding canceled appointments by following these steps.

- Click **Finish** to close the appointment book and return to the Reception desk. Click on **Policy** to open the office Policy Manual.
- Type "cancel" in the search bar and click the magnifying glass once to read the office policy regarding canceled appointments.

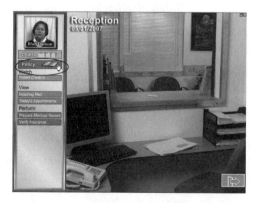

- Click **Close Manual** to return to the Reception desk.

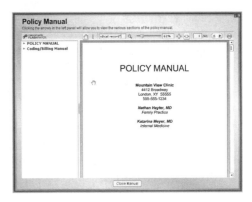

2. What is the role of the medical assistant in providing information about cancellations to the physician?

3. According to the Policy Manual, what is the next step to be taken with this patient who has canceled his last three appointments? Explain your answer.

Exercise 2

Writing Activity

15 minutes

1. Below, compose a letter to the patient you identified in question 1. In the letter, describe the reason for possible termination and the necessary steps needed to remain a patient of Dr. Meyer. The letter should include all of the reasons for possible termination and the need for the patient to keep appointments as made. The letter can also state that Dr. Meyer is concerned about continuity of care and the need for patient safety through this continuity of care.

Mountain View Clinic

4412 Broadway / London, XY 55555 / Phone: (555) 555-1234 / Fax: (555) 555-1239

Nathan Hayler, MD - Family Practice / Katarina Meyer, MD - Internal Medicine

2. Why does the letter need to be sent by certified mail?

Thought Question

3. If a decision is made to terminate a patient, how much time must be allowed between notification and the termination?

→ • Remain in the Reception area with Rhea Davison and continue to the next exercise.

Exercise 3

Online Activity—Maintaining Licensure and Credentials

 15 minutes

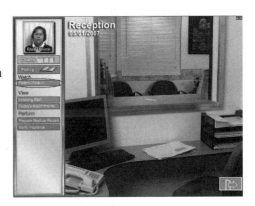

- At the Reception desk with Rhea Davison, click on **Patient Check-In** to view the video. (*Note:* If you have exited the program, sign in again to Mountain View Clinic, select Rhea Davison from the patient list, go to the Reception area, and view the video.)

- At the end of the video, click **Close**.

In the video, the medical assistant discusses the CMA(AAMA) credential. However, the RMA is another credential that is recognized on a national level. *Note:* The CMA credential must now be written as CMA(AAMA) to be distinguished from other CMA credentials that are not Certified Medical Assisting Credentials.

1. Look up the CMA(AAMA) and RMA credentials and name the organizations that award these credentials.

2. Research your state to see if there are any state or regional examinations or credentials awarded by area or region.

3. On arrival this morning, Dr. Meyer states that you need to check on the status of her renewed medical license because it has not arrived. She reminds you that her current license expires on June 1. Go to the Internet and find the name and address of the medical examining board for the state in which you live. Also find the time limit for medical licensure and any necessary components for renewal of the license. Print your findings for your instructor.

➡ • Remain in the Reception area and continue to the next exercise.

Exercise 4

Online Activity—Maintaining Confidentiality and Explaining Office Policy to the Patient

40 minutes

• This exercise continues with questions regarding the video of Rhea Davison's check-in. If you need to review the video again, click on **Patient Check-In** at the Reception desk. (*Note:* If you have exited the program, sign in again to Mountain View Clinic, select Rhea Davison from the patient list, go to the Reception area, and view the video again if necessary.)

1. Ms. Davison is an established patient. Did Kristin handle Ms. Davison's late arrival in a professional manner? Explain your answer.

2. Would you have expected Ms. Davison to be upset if her appointment had to be rescheduled?

3. What was your feeling about Kristin and the issue of confidentiality just before the arrival of the office manager?

4. The office manager appeared to be upset with Ms. Davison, but do you think she was more upset with Ms. Davison or with her employee Kristin?

5. The office manager explained the need to follow HIPAA policy and the need for confidentiality of medical records. How do you feel about the attitude of the office manager while discussing the matter of confidentiality?

6. Why does the office manager need to explain the HIPAA policy in such a specific manner?

Exercise 5

**Writing Activity—Obtaining Travel Itineraries and Locating Information
for the Physician**

 90 minutes

1. Prepare and provide a travel itinerary for one of the physicians at Mountain View Clinic, following these steps:
   a. Using the Internet as your tool, make travel arrangements for Dr. Meyer to attend the next American Association of Medical Assistants (AAMA) Conference. Dr. Meyer is scheduled to speak on Saturday afternoon at 4 p.m. and would like to arrive at the airport by noon that day. She plans to spend one night and would like a return flight on Sunday arriving no later than 7 p.m.
   b. Decide on the best flight to meet Dr. Meyer's needs from your site (your geographic location) of practice. Record the fare, times of departure and arrival, and any special identification or security requirements.
   c. Make arrangements for Dr. Meyer at the hotel where the conference is to be held, showing the room fee including taxes. Make a notation of the check-in time and the check-out time at the hotel.
   d. Finally, arrange for land transportation for Dr. Meyer from the airport to the hotel and back to the airport. Some hotels have a complimentary shuttle or can recommend a shuttle company. You can also check the price of renting a car or the approximate cost for taxi service.

2. Travel restrictions and requirements change frequently, particularly for travel outside of the United States. Using the Internet as a resource, locate websites that provide updated information on security, restrictions, and requirements for travelers.

3. Dr. Meyer is scheduled to present a speech on sleep apnea at the conference. She asks you to consult the Internet and find five links she can use as information resources as she prepares her speech. What did you find?

   (1)

   (2)

   (3)

   (4)

   (5)

Exercise 6

Writing Activity—Maintaining Liability Insurance

15 minutes

   1. Why is liability insurance important in the medical office?

2. What steps can the medical assistant take to protect patients from injury in the medical office? List five ways the medical assistant can reduce the chance of accidents.

3. Why is it important for the person responsible for liability insurance to keep a "tickler" file of the dates when premiums are due?

4. Can an electronic date reminder such as one on the Outlook Express calendar be utilized for this purpose to ensure that the premium is paid on time?

LESSON 2

Telephone Techniques

👓 **Reading Assignment:** Chapter 5—Interpersonal Skills and Human Behavior
  • The Process of Communication
  Chapter 9—Telephone Techniques

Patients: Louise Parlet, Wilson Metcalf

Learning Objectives:

- Describe how nonverbal and verbal communication skills are apparent when using the telephone.
- Understand the need for ethical and legal behavior on the telephone.
- Identify ways to ensure confidentiality when using the telephone in the medical office.
- Manage telephone calls professionally while handling other administrative duties.

Overview:

In this lesson, the legal and ethical issues related to the use of the telephone will be discussed. Issues of confidentiality when using the phone to make arrangements for transfer of a patient to an inpatient facility will also be covered. Proper telephone techniques are important in setting the mood for the entire office. This lesson is designed to provide basic understanding of these techniques.

30

Exercise 1

Online Activity—Proper Use of the Telephone in the Medical Office

40 minutes

- Sign in to Mountain View Clinic.
- From the patient list, select **Louise Parlet**.

- On the office map, highlight and click on **Reception** to enter the Reception area.

- Under the Watch heading, select **Patient Check-In** to view the video clip.

- At the end of the video, click **Close** to return to the Reception desk.

1. As Kristin answers the phone, how does she identify herself? Was her identification a correct procedure? Why or why not?

2. What nonverbal communication does Kristin convey when she answers the phone?

3. Kristin did not close the privacy window while talking on the telephone. Was this a break in confidentiality? Why or why not?

4. When should the privacy window be closed when the medical assistant is on the telephone?

5. Kristin stated "Please excuse me" so that she could answer the telephone. When she completed the phone call, she apologized for the interruption. Was this a proper telephone technique? Give a reason for your answer.

6. What was your opinion about the way the sales representative behaved while Ms. Parlet was at the counter?

7. Could Kristin have handled the sales representative's intrusion into their conversation in a more sensitive way from Ms. Parlet's perspective?

8. Assume that Kristin is engaged in a phone call that involves personal information about the medical condition of a patient. How can she determine whether she is communicating with a person to whom she can legally and ethically release the information?

- Click the exit arrow to go to the Summary Menu.
- On the Summary Menu, click **Return to Map**.

- From the patient list, select **Wilson Metcalf**.

- On the office map, highlight and click on **Check Out**.

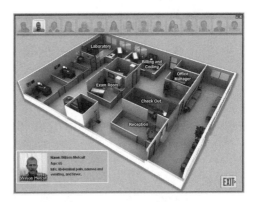

- Under the Watch heading, click on **Patient Check-Out** to view the video clip.

9. How is Mr. Metcalf's confidentiality safeguarded while the medical assistant is on the telephone?

10. How did the medical assistant verify the exact location of the patient transfer so that the orders could be sent as needed?

➤ • If you have not already closed the video, click **Close** to return to the Check Out desk.

• At the Check Out desk, click on **Charts** and then on the **Patient Information** tab. Select **7-Release of Information Authorization** from the drop-down menu.

11. Was it permissible for Leah to call Mr. Metcalf's son concerning his transfer to the hospital? Why or why not?

➤ • Go to the **Patient Information** tab again, and choose **1-Patient Information Form**. Look for Mr. Metcalf's son's telephone number.

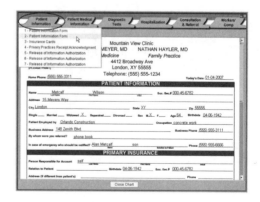

12. What telephone number was given for Mr. Metcalf's son Alan?

13. Would it have been better, in your opinion, to have Mr. Metcalf's son's phone number on the Release of Information Authorization? Why?

Exercise 2

Writing Activity

10 minutes

1. List different acceptable ways to introduce yourself if you were working at Mountain View Clinic, keeping in mind the rules for answering the phone that are discussed in your textbook. Practice each way out loud while holding the telephone. Choose which introduction seems most comfortable to you and be prepared to share your personal preference with your classmates.

3

Scheduling and Managing Appointments

/OFO **Reading Assignment:** Chapter 10—Scheduling Appointments

Patient: Janet Jones

Learning Objectives:

- Discuss the rationale for providing space in a day's appointment schedule for emergency appointments.
- Explain the need for a matrix on the appointment schedule.
- Describe the role of the Policy Manual in appointment scheduling.
- Explain the importance of verbal communication concerning appointment delays.
- Apply the skills of scheduling appointments.
- Apply the skills of maintaining the appointment book.
- Identify office policies concerning rescheduling appointments.
- Apply the skills of rescheduling appointments.

Overview:

In this lesson you will schedule and manage appointments using the policies established for this office. The patient, Janet Jones, is upset because she has not been seen immediately. You will discuss the proper way to deal with such a situation. After today's appointment, Janet Jones will need to come back for a follow-up appointment. You will schedule this appointment for her at the appropriate time.

Exercise 1

Online Activity—Using a Specific Daily Appointment Schedule

25 minutes

- Sign in to Mountain View Clinic
- From the patient list, select **Janet Jones**.

- On the office map, highlight and click on **Reception**.

- At the Reception desk, click **Today's Appointments** (under the View heading) to open the appointment book. Review the scheduled appointments, noting the time of Janet Jones' appointment. You will need to scroll down the appointment book to see the entire day.

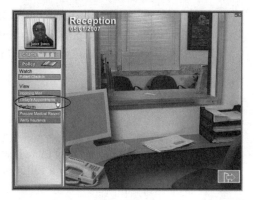

- Click **Finish** to close the appointment book and return to the Reception desk.

1. According to the appointment schedule, what time is Janet Jones' appointment?

2. If Janet Jones signed in at 1:30 p.m., would she have been on time for her appointment? Explain your answer.

- Under the Watch heading, click **Patient Check-In** and watch the video.
- Click **Close** at the end of the video to return to the Reception desk.

3. Janet Jones is upset when she arrives at the counter. How does Kristin handle the patient in a professional way through verbal and nonverbal communication?

4. Assuming that Ms. Jones checked in at 1:30 p.m., what would have been an appropriate statement for the receptionist to make as the patient checked in to prevent her from becoming so upset?

- At the Reception desk, click on **Policy** to open the office Policy Manual.

- Type "appointment scheduling" in the search bar and click once on the magnifying glass.
- Read the section of the Policy Manual on scheduling appointments and use this as a tool for answering the questions and scheduling the patient appointments.

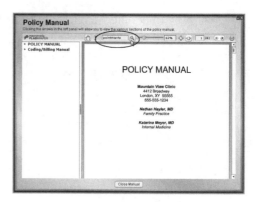

5. How much time is needed for an appointment during which a history and physical examination must be completed for a new patient?

6. Why is it necessary to set up a matrix before making appointments?

7. What buffer times are available for emergency appointments, and why is it important to have this time available?

8. According to the office Policy Manual, what would have been appropriate concerning rescheduling this patient's appointment?

9. Why is it important to identify Workers' Compensation appointments at the time of scheduling rather than at the time of the appointment?

10. Is the patient's time just as valuable as the physician's time?

→ • Click **Close Manual** to return to the Reception desk.
  • Leave **Reception** by clicking the exit arrow at the lower right corner of the screen.

  • At the Summary Menu, select **Return to Map** and continue to the next exercise.

Exercise 2

Writing Activity—Adding Appointments to a Schedule

20 minutes

At the end of the day on April 31, a list of patients needing appointments on May 1 was shown to Dr. Hayler and Dr. Meyer. Both physicians stated that because few patients were currently in the hospital, they would be able to see patients in the clinic earlier than usual the next morning. Dr. Hayler and Dr. Meyer will begin seeing patients at 8:15 a.m. The staff has been informed of the early start. The white areas of the appointment book indicate buffer times for adding patients who need to see the doctor today or for those patients with emergent needs. You may choose a patient, go to the Reception desk, open the Policy Manual, and type "appointment scheduling" in the search bar to review the length of time you will need to block off for each appointment.

1. a. Insert the following appointments for Dr. Hayler into the morning schedule on the next page.

    (1) Robert Leuker is a patient who has not been to the clinic in 5 years and wants to be seen for a lump in his arm. He has a past history of cancer and needs to be seen ASAP. He should be seen first in the morning so that he can be referred as necessary. He is insured through BlueCross/BlueShield (BC/BS). His phone number is (555) 555-8890.

    (2) Lindsey Repp needs a follow-up appointment for an earache and recurrent fever. She is insured through Central Health HMO and can be double-booked at the end of the appointment for Louise Parlet. Her telephone number is (555) 555-9004.

    (3) John Price, who needs a follow-up appointment for his blood pressure, has Medicare. His blood pressure was low when he took it yesterday, and he feels dizzy. He simply wants Dr. Hayler to reevaluate his medication. He can be seen just before lunch. Mr. Price's phone number is (555) 555-1998.

   b. After completing Dr. Hayler's appointments, add the following appointments for Dr. Meyer in the morning, using the same schedule on the next page.

    (1) Catherine Lake needs a follow-up appointment for pyelonephritis. She forgot to make her follow-up appointment when she was last seen. Ms. Lake is going out of town for 2 weeks and needs to see Dr. Meyer before leaving. Her insurance coverage is through BC/BS. Dr. Meyer will see her at the earliest appointment time. Catherine Lake's phone number is (555) 555-1865.

    (2) Lucille Meryl needs to be seen for a follow-up to a thyroid test. Dr. Meyer wants to see her as a double-booking at the end of the appointment for Rhea Davison. Her insurance is through Drake. Her phone number is (555) 555-3219.

    (3) An established patient, Simon Reed, calls at 11:30 a.m. to tell you that he has some chest pain, and even though he has an appointment for tomorrow, he does not think he should wait. Mr. Reed has experienced a heart attack in the past. When you discuss this with Dr. Meyer, she tells you to phone 911 while keeping the patient on the line. She also says that she will go to the hospital to see Mr. Reed once he is in the Emergency Department. What notation should you make on the schedule?

5/1/2007	Dr. Hayler			Dr. Meyer	
	Patient Name	Insurance		Patient Name	Insurance
8:00 AM	(Hospital rounds) Joe Smitty - Chem 12, CBC Marsha Brady - Fasting BS			(Hospital rounds)	
8:15 AM	(Hospital rounds)			(Hospital rounds) Joanne Crosby, PT, PTT (555) 555-1865	
8:30 AM	Louise Parlet, Est. Pt. New Pregnancy/Pelvic (555) 555-3214	Teachers		Rhea Davison, Est. Pt. Elevated BS, abdominal distention, pelvic (555) 555-5656	None
8:45 AM					
9:00 AM					
9:15 AM					
9:30 AM				Hu Huang, Est. Pt. Severe cough, fever (555) 555-1464	Medicare
9:45 AM	Jade Wong, NP 7 mos well child checkup / immunization (555) 555-3345	Central Health HMO			
10:00 AM				Chris O'Neil back pain (pt. cancelled - resched 5/7) Jesus Santo, Walk-in Leg pain, SOB	None
10:15AM					
10:30 AM				Jean Deere, Est. Pt. Memory loss, ear pain (555) 555-6361	Medicare
10:45 AM	Tristan Tsosie, Est. Pt. Suture Removal (555) 555-1515	Blue Cross / Blue Shield			
11:00 AM					
11:15 AM				Wilson Metcalf, Est. Pt. N/V, abdominal pain, difficulty urinating - (555) 555-3311	Medicare
11:30 AM	LUNCH				
11:45 AM					
12:00 PM					
12:15 PM	Renee Anderson, NP Annual GYN Exam (555) 555-3331	Blue Cross / Blue Shield			

2. You must now call John Price to inform him that Dr. Hayler will see him just before lunch. Write the information below that Mr. Price will need to be told. Why did Dr. Hayler need to be contacted before making the appointment for Mr. Price?

3. You must also call Lucille Meryl to inform her that Dr. Meyer wants to see her about her test results. What information do you need to provide, and how would you answer her when she questions why she needs to be seen so quickly?

Exercise 3

Online Activity—Preparing an Appointment Schedule

30 minutes

- In this exercise we will continue with Janet Jones' visit. If you are already at the office map, click on **Check Out** to go to the Check Out desk. (*Note:* If you have exited the program, sign in again to Mountain View Clinic, select Janet Jones, and go to the Check Out desk.)
- At the Check Out desk, click **Encounter Form** under the View heading.

1. At what date should Janet Jones return to the clinic for a follow-up appointment?

2. How much time should be allotted to the follow-up appointment for Ms. Jones?

 • Click **Finish** to return to Check Out.
- Click **Patient Check Out** under the Watch heading.

3. At what time of day was Ms. Jones follow-up appointment made?

Complete the following activities using the appointment sheets on the next two pages.

(1) Set up the appointment sheet for the date that Janet Jones is to return for her follow-up visit at the same time the medical assistant in the video scheduled her appointment.

(2) Using the information in the Policy Manual, set up the matrix for that day. (*Note:* If you need to review this, return to the Policy Manual, type "hours of operation" in the search bar, and click once on the magnifying glass.)

(3) Add an appointment at 11:00 a.m. for Kay Soto (an established patient) with Dr. Meyer. Ms. Soto has been prescribed a weight loss program and is coming in for a weight check. Her insurance is through Metro HMO. Ms. Soto's phone number is (555) 555-0954.

(4) George Smith, age 15, is to be seen by Dr. Hayler for a football injury the night before. He has State Agricultural Insurance and is an existing patient. George needs to be seen as early as possible so that he can go to school. Mr. Smith's phone number is (555) 555-8778.

(5) Callie Agree, a new patient, is to be seen for a possible sinus infection. She has Medicare and will be accompanied by her daughter. The daughter prefers to see Dr. Meyer in the midmorning so that her mother will have time to dress. Ms. Agree's phone number is (555) 555-3452.

(6) Sophie Coats, age 6 months, is an established patient who will be seen by Dr. Hayler for a well-baby visit. She is due to have immunizations at this visit. Her mother prefers to have an appointment as early in the morning as possible. Sophie is covered by her father's insurance with Banker's Health. Ms. Coats' phone number is (555) 554-0090.

(7) Mamie Mack, age 18, is an established patient who needs a physical examination for college. She prefers to be seen by Dr. Hayler. Either late morning or early afternoon is better for her since she is still in school. She is covered through George Allen Insurance at her mother's place of employment. Ms. Mack's phone number is (555) 554-8745.

(8) Kay Soto calls to cancel her appointment for the day because she has to leave town to take care of her ill mother. She does not want to reschedule at this time.

(9) Dr. Hayler will need to leave at 11:15 a.m. for a dental appointment but will be back in the afternoon. Mark this on the appointment sheet.

(10) Dr. Meyer is scheduled to be off the afternoon of this day. Mark this on the appointment sheet.

4.

/ /2007	Dr. Hayler		Dr. Meyer	
Time	Patient Name	Insurance	Patient Name	Insurance
8:00 AM				
8:15 AM				
8:30 AM				
8:45 AM				
9:00 AM				
9:15 AM				
9:30 AM				
9:45 AM				
10:00 AM				
10:15 AM				
10:30 AM				
10:45 AM				
11:00 AM				
11:15 AM				
11:30 AM				
11:45 AM				
12:00 PM				
12:15 PM				

5.

/ /2007	Dr. Hayler			Dr. Meyer		
Time	Patient Name		Insurance	Patient Name		Insurance
12:30 PM						
12:45 PM						
1:00 PM						
1:15 PM						
1:30 PM						
1:45 PM						
2:00 PM						
2:15 PM						
2:30 PM						
2:45 PM						
3:00 PM						
3:15 PM						
3:30 PM						
3:45 PM						
4:00 PM						
4:15 PM						
4:30 PM						
4:45 PM						
5:00 PM						

6. Which is the necessary procedure for canceling Kay Soto's appointment?
   a. Erase the canceled appointment and tell Ms. Soto that there will be a charge because she did not give 24 hours notice.
   b. Cross out the appointment (using the office-preferred writing implement) and record the cancellation in the patient medical record.
   c. Report the cancellation to Dr. Meyer.
   d. Tell her that she must reschedule this appointment today for continued medical care.

LESSON 4 _____

Scheduling Admissions and Procedures

Reading Assignment: Chapter 10—Scheduling Appointments
- Scheduling Other Types of Appointments

Chapter 14—The Paper Medical Record
- Releasing Medical Record Information

Patients: Wilson Metcalf, Shaunti Begay

Learning Objectives:

- Recognize the patient information that needs to be sent to a medical facility if your office is making a referral.
- Check the patient's records to verify who is authorized by the patient to receive information regarding the patient.
- Use the Policy Manual to determine the responsibility of the medical assistant in making arrangements for inpatient admissions and referrals to other physicians.
- Explain why it is important to arrange outpatient appointments at a time convenient for the patient.
- Recognize confidentiality issues that must be followed when making arrangements to transfer a patient to a hospital.

Overview:

In this lesson you will make the necessary arrangements for moving Wilson Metcalf from the office to the hospital. You will ensure that his family has been notified of the move. With Shaunti Begay, you will make arrangements for outpatient testing and schedule an office appointment for providing her test results. This patient will also need to see a specialist, so any questions concerning the insurance for these appointments will need to be answered.

Exercise 1

Online Activity—Scheduling Inpatient Admissions and Procedures

30 minutes

- Sign in to Mountain View Clinic.
- From the patient list, select **Wilson Metcalf**.

- On the office map, highlight and click on **Check Out**.

- Click on **Policy** to open the office Policy Manual.
- Type "job description" in the search bar and click once on the magnifying glass.
- Read the section of the Policy Manual concerning the job descriptions for the medical assistants.

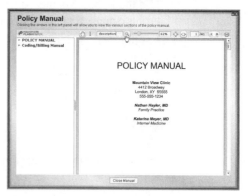

1. According to office policy, which medical assistant has the primary duty of making the arrangements for inpatient admissions and for making referrals to other physicians?

- Click **Close Manual** to return to the Check Out desk.
- Under the Watch heading, select **Patient Check-Out** to view the video. At the end of the video, click **Close**.

2. Which documents are being copied and sent to the hospital with Mr. Metcalf according to the video? Select all that apply.

_____ Medicare card

_____ Private insurance card

_____ Authorization form

_____ Office registration

_____ Physician's orders

- Click on **Charts** to open Wilson Metcalf's medical record.
- Next, click on the **Patient Information** tab and select **3-Insurance Cards** from the drop-down menu.

- Click again on the **Patient Information** tab, select **1-Patient Information Form**, and review this form.

- Once again, click on the **Patient Information** tab. Select **6-Release of Information Authorization Form** from the drop-down menu.
- Note that both the Patient Information Form and the Release of Information Authorization Form are dated 5-1-2007.
- Click **Close Chart** when you have finished reviewing the documents.

3. Why would it be appropriate to send the office registration and authorization form to the hospital for Wilson Metcalf's admission?

4. Who may receive information concerning Mr. Metcalf's medical condition? Can the entire medical record be released?

5. Did Leah act within the ethical and legal boundaries to release the information she gave to the hospital for Mr. Metcalf? Explain your answer.

6. Why is it important that the window to the waiting room be closed while Leah is making arrangements for Mr. Metcalf to be transferred to the hospital?

Exercise 2

Online Activity—Scheduling Outpatient Admissions and Procedures

20 minutes

- From the patient list, select **Shaunti Begay**. (*Note:* If you have exited the program, sign in again to Mountain View Clinic and select Shaunti Begay from the patient list.)

- Highlight and click on **Check Out** on the office map.

- Select **Charts** to open Shaunti Begay's medical record.

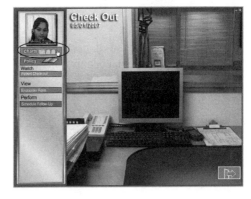

- Under the **Patient Medical Information** tab, select **2-Progress Notes** to read the documentation on the current visit.

1. What appointments does the medical assistant who is checking patients out need to make?

 • Click **Close Chart**.
- Under the Watch heading, select **Patient Check-Out** to view the video.

- When you have finished watching the video, click **Close**.

2. Did Leah make sure the referral for outpatient admission and procedures was scheduled at a time convenient for the patient and her family?

3. Why is it important to check that referrals and appointments to specialists are made at a time that is convenient for the patient?

4. Shaunti's father, Mr. Begay, is concerned with the financial aspects of the visit because his insurance is not a provider for this medical office. Leah provided the information about his insurance carrier and the referral. However, she did not provide information that was needed to assist Shaunti in the referral. Can you name two items that were not discussed with Mr. Begay or given to Mr. Begay?

5. Refer back to the Progress Notes and then look at the referral authorization in Shaunti's chart; compare it with the Progress Notes. Did Leah gain approval for all the tests the doctor wants the patient to have?

6. Mr. Begay was concerned about the amount of the bill for Shaunti. Do you think that Leah was professional in her handling of verbal and nonverbal communication in this interaction? In what way, if any, would you have changed what was said or done? Did Leah act in an ethical manner?

→ • From the Check Out area, click on **Encounter Form** (under the View heading). Review this form.

• Next, under the Perform heading, click on **Schedule Follow-Up**.

• Complete the checklist and click **Finish**.

• Click on the exit arrow at the bottom of the screen to leave the area.

• On the Summary Menu, select **Look at Your Performance Summary** to compare your answers with those of the experts.

• You may save and print the performance summary for your records or to turn in to your instructor.

Maintaining a Proper Inventory

∽ **Reading Assignment:** Chapter 12—The Office Environment and Daily Operations
- Supplies and Equipment in the Physician's Office

Patients: None

Learning Objectives:

- Describe the steps necessary for replenishing supplies.
- Discuss how having too many or too few supplies can affect the efficiency of the office.
- Decide which items to reorder and the amount to reorder.
- Explain the necessity of checking equipment for maintenance on a regular basis.
- Discuss the role of the medical assistant in suggesting new equipment for the medical office.
- Describe the proper disposal of controlled substances that are found to be out of date.

Overview:

Ensuring the availability of supplies and equipment when needed is essential to maintaining the efficiency of the medical office practice. The proper inventory of supplies and equipment helps to ensure their availability. In some cases, it is more efficient to order supplies in larger quantities. The medical assistant also has the responsibility of making sure that the equipment ordered is the most currently used in the field. Finally, when medications are found to be out of date, proper disposal is necessary. This lesson will focus on supplies and equipment and their importance to office efficiency.

Exercise 1

Online Activity—Deciding When to Replenish Supplies

🕐 30 minutes

- Sign in to Mountain View Clinic.
- On the office map, highlight and click on **Office Manager** to enter the manager's office. (*Note:* You do not need to select a patient for this exercise.)

- Click on **Supply Inventory** to view the inventory records.

- To view the record for each item in the inventory, click on the corresponding tab headings.

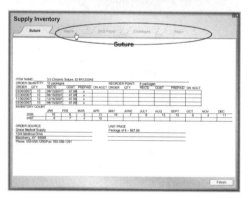

1. What is the reorder point for sutures?

2. Looking at the record from 2006, how many packages of sutures were previously used in May?

Copyright © 2011, 2007 by Saunders, an imprint of Elsevier Inc. All rights reserved.

→ • Click on the tab heading for **Gauze** to view the inventory record.

3. What is the reorder point for gauze?

4. Looking at the record from 2006, how many bags of gauze were previously used in May?

5. The inventory for gauze is recorded as bags, but gauze can also be ordered by the case. How many bags are in one case?

6. What is the unit price? Does this represent the price per bag or the price per case?

7. What is the discount offered for ordering four or more cases of gauze?

8. After looking at the inventory supply sheet for gauze, should gauze be reordered? If so, why and how much? If not, why not? If you reorder, what will be the net amount of the purchase?

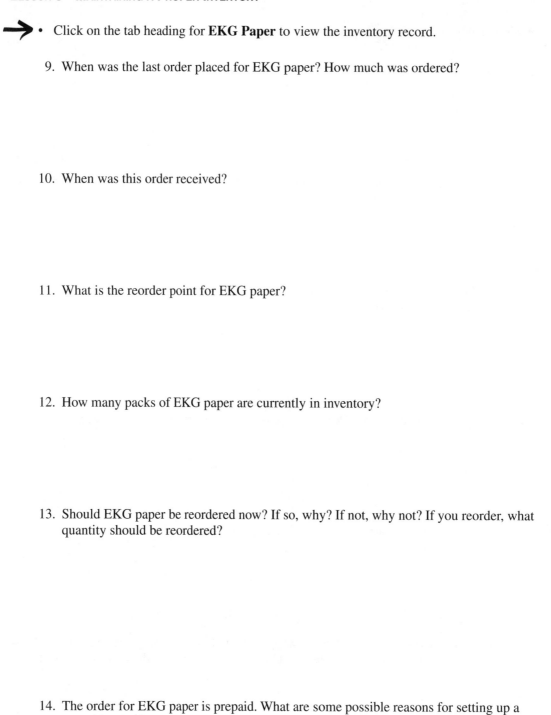

→ • Click on the tab heading for **EKG Paper** to view the inventory record.

9. When was the last order placed for EKG paper? How much was ordered?

10. When was this order received?

11. What is the reorder point for EKG paper?

12. How many packs of EKG paper are currently in inventory?

13. Should EKG paper be reordered now? If so, why? If not, why not? If you reorder, what quantity should be reordered?

14. The order for EKG paper is prepaid. What are some possible reasons for setting up a prepaid order for this item?

→ • Click on the tab heading for **Envelopes** to view the inventory record.

15. How often does the office normally order envelopes?

16. On February 28, 2007, the office ordered four more boxes of envelopes. When did this order arrive?

17. Why is there so much time between when the order is placed and when the order is received?

18. From what you see on the inventory form, do the envelopes need to be reordered? How could the office lower the price of the envelopes? Do you see a problem with the reorder point, and does this need to be changed? If the envelopes should be reordered in bulk, what would be the price?

→ • Click on the tab heading for **Paper** to view the inventory record for copier paper.

19. After examining the inventory supply card for copier paper, what is the cost for three cases?

20. What is the cost for ordering five cases?

21. Below, fill out the purchase order for three cases of copier paper. The shipping fee is $6.00 and the sales tax is 6%.

Office Station

Purchase Order

Bill To:
Mountain View Clinic
4412 Broadway
London, XY 55555

Ship To:
Mountain View Clinic
4412 Broadway
London, XY 55555

Order #:
Date:

Delivery Required By:

Sales Contact	Terms	Tax ID

Item	Quantity	Description	Unit Price	Disc %	Total

Shipping	
Subtotal	
Tax %	
Balance Due	

145 Oceanus Way, St. Pinot, XY 53559
Phone: (123) 456 7890 Fax: (123) 456 7899 CSR@officestation.com

Office Station

INVOICE # 2297

DATE:
Customer Name: Mountain View Clinic

BILL TO:		SHIP TO:	
COMPANY NAME: Mountain View Clinic		COMPANY NAME: Mountain View Clnic	
COMPANY ADDRESS: 4412 Broadway London, XY 55555		COMPANY ADDRESS: 4412 Broadway London, XY 55555	

Order #	Sales Contact	Terms	Tax ID
105699			

Item	Quantity	Description	Unit Price	Disc %	Total
CPO-117	3 cases	Copier Paper	$71.27 / 3 cases		$71.27

Shipping	$6.00
Subtotal	$77.27
Tax %	$4.64
Balance Due	$81.91

145 Oceanus Way, St. Pinot, XY 53559
Phone: (123) 456 7890   Fax: (123) 456 7899   CSR@officestation.com

22. Using the information on the invoice above, complete the check on the next page to pay for the delivered supplies.

173980

DATE: _____

TO: _____

FOR: _____

ACCOUNT NO. _____

AMOUNT PAID $ _____

MOUNTAIN VIEW CLINIC
4412 Broadway
London, XY 55555

Date: _____

173980

94-724.224

Pay to the order of: _____

_____ Dollars $ _____

Clarion National Bank
Member FDIC
90 Grape Vine Road
London, XY 55555-0001

Authorized Signature

||⬛ 005503 ||⬛ 446782011 ||⬛ 678800470

23. How should the ordered supplies be handled when they arrive at the office?

Exercise 2

Writing Activity—Properly Disposing Medications

🕐 10 minutes

- Sign in to Mountain View Clinic and select any patient from the patient list.
- On the office map, highlight and click on **Reception** to enter the Reception area.
- Click on **Policy** to open the office Policy Manual.
- Type "medications" in the search bar and click once on the magnifying glass.
- Read the section of the Policy Manual concerning the office policy in regard to the disposal of medications.

1. While checking supplies, Cathy notices that some of the nonscheduled medications are out of date. These medications are oral tablets and capsules. What means of disposal is correct for these medications?

2. If part of a schedule II medication ampule has to be disposed of, how many clinical medical assistants need to witness the disposal?

Exercise 3

Writing Activity—Maintaining Administrative Equipment

10 minutes

1. When filling the copier with paper, Cathy notices that it is time for regular maintenance of the machine and the representative has not been to the office. According to the Policy Manual, the office manager is responsible for maintaining the facilities. What should Cathy's next step be?

2. The toner cartridges are low, and Cathy sees a need for replenishing these. What should she do?

Exercise 4

Writing Activity—Suggestions for Equipment and Supplies

10 minutes

1. Ameeta has observed that not all patients with diabetes are using the same glucose meters at home. The physicians are asking that quality control be checked with patients more often. However, if the office does not have the same glucometers and supplies that some of the patients use at home, it is difficult to provide accurate patient teaching. What steps should Ameeta take to ensure that patient teaching is accurate and helpful for each patient?

2. Leah, as an administrative assistant, has found that the phone line for the fax machine is often busy when a fax needs to be received. Often the person attempting to send the fax has called to complain of the difficulty of getting important information to the physicians. What steps should Leah take to show the need for another fax line for the hospital?

Written Communications

6

Reading Assignment: Chapter 13—Written Communication and Mail Processing

Patient: Wilson Metcalf

Learning Objectives:

- Prepare letters in response to the mail received.
- Use correct grammar, spelling, and formatting techniques in letter writing.
- Read mail correspondence correctly.

Overview:

In this lesson you will be asked to respond to incoming mail that includes an NSF check and a letter from a collection agency.

Exercise 1

Online Activity—Reading Mail and Composing a Letter for an NSF Check

40 minutes

- Sign in to Mountain View Clinic.
- From the patient list, select **Wilson Metcalf**.

- On the office map, highlight and click on **Reception** to enter the Reception area.

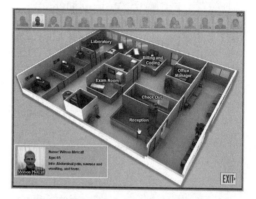

- Under the View heading, select **Incoming Mail** to view the mail received by the clinic.
- Click the numbers to examine and read each piece of mail.

1. Were any payments received in the mail today?

2. List the people from whom payments were received.

➡ 3. What is the name of the physician who sent a consultation letter to Dr. Meyer?

4. Who was the letter in reference to?

➡ • From the list of mail at the top of the screen, click on **7** to view that piece of mail again.
   • Leave the Incoming Mail window open as you complete the remaining exercises.

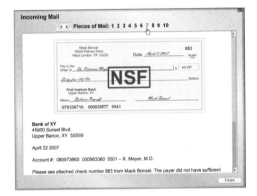

5. On the next page, write your letter to the patient about the NSF check, using an acceptable format. Be sure your message conveys the need to handle this matter within a certain number of days. Also inform the patient that no further checks will be accepted for this patient's medical care at Mountain View Clinic. This should be prepared for a signature by the office manager.

Mountain View Clinic

4412 Broadway / London, XY 55555 / Phone: (555) 555-1234 / Fax (555) 555-1239

Nathan Hayler, MD - Family Practice / Katarina Meyer, MD - Internal Medicine

Exercise 2

Online Activity—Composing a Letter in Response to an Inaccurate Accounts Payable

30 minutes

- From the list of mail at the top of the screen, click on **10** to read the letter from Summer Oxygen Company.
- Click **Finish** to return to the Reception Desk.

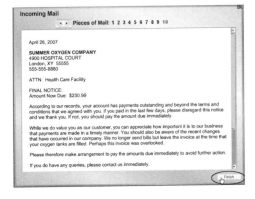

- Click the exit arrow to leave the Reception area.
- On the Summary Menu, click **Return to Map**.

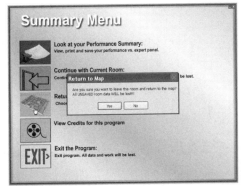

- On the office map, highlight and click on **Office Manager** to enter the manager's office.

- Under the View heading, click on **Bank Statement** to view the most recent statement from the bank.

• Select the **Check Ledger** tab to review the most recent checks written by Mountain View Clinic.

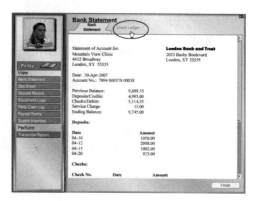

1. There was a payment made to Summer Oxygen Company for $230.99.

   a. According to the check ledger, what was the date the payment was made?

   b. What was the check number?

• Click on the **Bank Statement** tab to review the account activity for April 2007.

2. Did check #1230 for $230.99 clear the account, according to the bank statement?

• Click **Finish** to return to the manager's office.

3. Below, compose a letter to the oxygen supply company in response to the claim that the invoice has not been paid. Write your letter using an acceptable format. Be sure your message includes all information needed to clear the accounts payable. This should be prepared for signature by the office manager.

Mountain View Clinic

4412 Broadway / London, XY 55555 / Phone: (555) 555-1234 / Fax (555) 555-1239

Nathan Hayler, MD - Family Practice / Katarina Meyer, MD - Internal Medicine

LESSON 7

Organizing a Patient's Medical Record

───

✎ **Reading Assignment:** Chapter 14—The Paper Medical Record
- Creating an Efficient Medical Records Management System
- Organization of the Medical Record
- Contents of the Complete Case History
- Making Additions to the Patient Record
- Keeping Records Current

Chapter 15—The Electronic Medical Record
- Executive Order to Promote Interoperability of EMR Systems
- Technological Terms in Health Information

Patients: Renee Anderson, Tristan Tsosie

Learning Objectives:

- Discuss why proper organization of the medical record is essential.
- Identify and describe the forms found in a medical record.
- Apply principles of medical record organization to choose forms that would be needed when preparing a new patient's medical record.
- Determine if forms need to be added to the medical record for an established patient.
- Describe the appropriate care of a damaged medical record.
- Determine the appropriate division of medical records when a new record must be established.
- Understand the difference between the terms Electronic Health Record (EHR), Electronic Medical Record (EMR), and Personal Health Record (PHR).
- Identify the goal of EMR interoperability.

Overview:

In this lesson we will explore the importance of preparing a patient's medical record correctly. Because the medical record is a legal document that shows the chronological care of the patient, this document must be correctly organized to ensure that information can be located as needed. Incorrectly organized charts not only cause frustration, but also decrease the efficiency of the medical practice. In this lesson you will organize a medical record for a new patient. For an

75

established patient, you will ensure that information received from other sources has been properly organized and that the information is readily available when the patient arrives for an appointment. You will also be asked to distinguish between the terms Electronic Medical Records and Electronic Health Records.

Exercise 1

Online Activity—Organizing a Medical Record for a New Patient

30 minutes

- Sign in to Mountain View Clinic.
- From the patient list, select **Renee Anderson**.

- Highlight and click on **Reception** on the office map.

- Click on **Policy** to open the Policy Manual. In the search bar, type "medical record" and click on the magnifying glass to search.

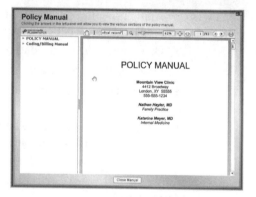

- Scroll up and down to read the duties assigned to the various types of medical assistants in the office.

1. At Mountain View Clinic, the Policy Manual states that the _____ medical assistant is responsible for preparing and organizing the medical record.

2. Why is it important for the administrative medical assistant to provide the necessary forms in a medical record for a new patient?

3. Follow the directions below to assemble a medical record. Your selections will be compared against those of an expert during the Performance Summary.

- When you have finished reading the relevant policy, click on **Close Manual** to return to the Reception desk.

- At the Reception desk, click on **Prepare Medical Record** (under the Perform heading) to begin assembling a chart for Ms. Anderson's visit.

- Next, go to Assemble Medical Record and click on **Perform** to begin selecting the forms necessary for Ms. Anderson's visit.

- The Patient Information tab is automatically chosen as the starting point when you access the Assemble Medical Record screen. Under Forms Available, choose the forms that should be filed under the Patient Information tab. Click **Add** to complete your selections. (*Note:* To select multiple consecutive forms, hold down the Shift key while making your selections. To make multiple nonconsecutive selections, hold down the Control [Ctrl] key as you click on your choices.) If you change your mind about a form you have added to a tab, click to highlight the name of the form and then click on **Remove** at the bottom of the screen.

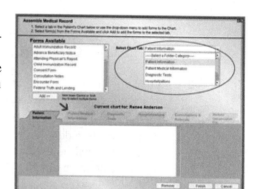

- Make note of which forms you add in the space below.

- When you have completed the Patient Information section, continue adding forms to the appropriate tabs in Renee Anderson's medical record. To select a new tab, either click on the tab on the medical record itself or use the drop-down menu to the right of Select Chart Tab.

- If you change you mind about a form you have added to a tab, click to highlight the name of the form and then click **Remove** at the bottom of the screen.

- When you are satisfied that you have selected all the necessary forms and put them in the correct tab sections, click **Finish** to close the medical record.

- Now click on the exit arrow at the bottom of screen to leave the Reception area.

- On the Summary Menu, click on **Look at Your Performance Summary** to compare your answers against those of the experts. How did you do?

- The icons for saving and printing the Performance Summary are located at the top right corner of the screen. (*Note:* If you do not save your Performance Summary, all data will be lost when you return to the map.)

- Click **Close**.
- Click **Return to Map**.

4. The form that contains the patient's demographic information is the

_____.

5. The form in the medical record that contains subjective information about the patient's

illnesses in the past is the _____.

6. The legal document that must be signed to allow information to be used to file insurance is

the _____.

7. The form used at each visit that allows the physician to record findings in the medical

record is the _____.

Exercise 2

Online Activity—Determining Whether to Add Forms to the Medical Record of an Established Patient

20 minutes

- From the patient list, click on **Tristan Tsosie**. (*Note:* If you have exited the program, sign in again to Mountain View Clinic and select Tristan Tsosie from the patient list.)

- On the office map, click on **Reception**.
- At the Reception desk, click on **Charts**.
- Click on the **Hospitalization** tab. From the drop-down menu, select **1-ED Record**.
- Read the ED Record to decide what other forms should be available for the physician for this office visit and to determine whether Tristan is following the orders of the physician who saw him in the Emergency Department. Think about which procedures the patient had while at the Emergency Department and which procedure should have a report to be filed in his chart. Then look under the tabs to see if you can find the report that you would also need to have available for the physician.
- Click on **Close Chart** to return to the Reception area.
- Under the Perform heading, select **Prepare Medical Record**.
- Click on the **Perform** button next to Review and Update Medical Records.

• Check the forms in each chart tab to be sure that the needed information for this visit is located under the correct tab and will be available when the physician needs it. Add any forms that you think are needed for this visit. If you think it is necessary, you may also remove or move any forms within the chart. (*Note:* If you need help with these steps, see the detailed instructions in Exercise 1 of this lesson.)

• When you are done, click **Finish** and then click the exit arrow to leave the Reception area.

• On the Summary Menu, click **Look at Your Performance Summary**.

All of the forms were in the chart that will be needed for Tristan's visit. His ED report and the radiology report were in his health record.

1. Explain the difference between the terms Electronic Medical Record (EMR) and Electronic Health Records (EHR).

2. If the medical office were sharing information with the hospital, would the record be called EMR or EHR?

3. Did the Emergency Department report advise the patient of when (number of days) to follow up with the doctor? Could this omission of information lead to problems with the patient's follow-up care?

4. Was (were) the report(s), other than the ED Record, available in the record?

5. When adding a report to the medical record, the medical assistant should:
   a. be sure the physician has seen the report before filing it.
   b. place the forms in the medical record in chronological order, with the earliest record on top.
   c. always be sure the date of arrival has been stamped on the form.
   d. wait to file the form just before the patient's arrival for an appointment.
   e. do both a and d.

6. When the medical assistant files materials in the medical record of an established patient, the materials should be filed in what order?

7. When accessing Tristan's medical record on arrival, you notice that the forms from the hospital have been torn during transmittal. What steps do you need to take to protect the record from further damage?

8. If a patient's folder is old, torn, or simply worn, what should the medical assistant do?

9. If a chart is overcrowded and a second chart needs to be established, how far back should the records that are moved to the new chart go? How should the record be marked to show that more than one medical record is available?

10. If the medical office is using an EMR that is interoperable with the hospital's EMR, would the physician have been able to access Tristan's records without having a paper copy in the medical record?

11. What is the goal of EMR interoperability?

12. Who manages, shares, and has control of the information in the Personal Health Record (PHR)?

LESSON 8

Filing Medical Records

Reading Assignment: Chapter 14—The Paper Medical Record
- Creating an Efficient Medical Records Management System
- Filing Procedures
- Filing Methods
- Organization of Files

Chapter 15—The Electronic Medical Record
- Technological Terms in Health Information
- Capabilities of EMR Systems

Patients: All

Learning Objectives:

- Alphabetize patient names for efficiency in filing medical records.
- List the necessary steps needed to prepare a paper medical record for filing.
- Describe the use of color coding to enhance paper medical record systems.
- Identify the filing systems used most frequently in the medical office for patient records.
- Discuss the differences between alphabetic and numeric filing systems.
- Determine which patients are established patients and which are new patients for preparing charts.
- Discuss the means for finding displaced paper medical records.
- Explain the most important function of primary features that EMR software may offer.

Overview:

Proper filing of medical records is essential in providing continuity of care for patients. You will determine if patients are new or established in preparation for filing and you will then alphabetize patients. You will be asked to differentiate between alphabetic and numeric filing systems and identify methods for locating misplaced medical information. One activity will involve answering questions about the different features with which typical EMR software comes.

Exercise 1

Online Activity—Preparing Patient Medical Records for Filing

50 minutes

- Sign in to Mountain View Clinic.
- One at a time, select each patient from the patient list across the top of the page (moving from left to right) and record his or her name in the table in question 1 below.

1. Record the names of all of the Mountain View Clinic patients in the first and third columns of the table below. Fill in all of column 1 first; then continue at the top of column 3.

Patient Name	First Date of Service; Last Date of Service	Patient Name	First Date of Service; Last Date of Service

• Now click again on any patient in the patient list. Then on the office map, click on **Reception**. At the Reception desk, click on **Today's Appointments** to view the day's schedule. Look for each patient's name and note next to his or her name in the table in question 1 whether that patient is a new patient (NP) or an established patient (Est. Pt.) (*Note:* You will return to fill in the remaining columns of the table later in this exercise.)

2. With the schedule of Today's Appointments still open, make a list below of the patients Dr. Hayler is to see in the morning. Place these patients in the correct order for their appointments and note whether the medical record can be pulled from the files of established patients or whether a new record should be prepared.

3. What medical records will need to be pulled from the files for Dr. Meyer's morning patients? Will any of these patients need to have a new record prepared? List these patients and their record needs below (in the order of their appointment times).

 • Click **Finish** to close the appointment book and return to the Reception desk.
 • Click the exit arrow in right lower corner of screen.

• From the Summary Menu, click on **Return to Map**; then click **Yes** to return to the office map and select another patient.

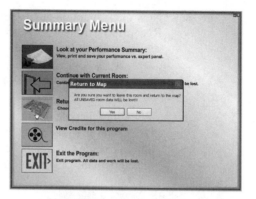

• Beginning with the first patient on the left in the patient list, click on **Reception**. Open the patient's chart, click on the **Patient Medical Information** tab, and select **Progress Notes**. Based on what you find, record the patient's first and last dates of service in columns 2 and 4 in the table in question 1.

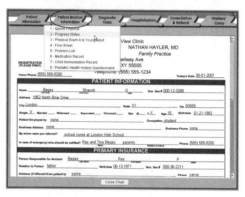

Important: New patients will not have any forms in their chart. Use today's virtual date—5-1-07—as their first date of service; there will be no "last date of service" for new patients.

• When you have recorded the date(s) for the first patient, click **Close Chart**; then click the exit arrow.
• From the Summary Menu, click on **Return to Map**.
• Select your next patient, open the chart, and record the date(s) in the table.
• Continue these steps for each patient until you have completed the table in question 1.

4. Using the table in question 1 as a reference, list the patients' names in alphabetic order in the left column below. In the right column indicate whether the medical records for each patient will be available in the file cabinet of established patients or whether the record will have to be organized and placed in the correct position as a new medical record.

Alphabetic List of Patients	New or Established Record?

5. As you pull the medical records for established patients, you will need to change the year on the medical records for these patients (unless the patient has already been seen in the current year). List the established patients below and indicate what year will need to be relabeled on their medical record (if this applies). Remember, today's virtual date is May 1, 2007.

Name of Established Patient	Year That Will Need to Be Relabeled

6. At the end of the morning, the medical records need to be filed correctly to prevent loss and to ensure proper time management. Below, list in alphabetic order the names of patients who had morning appointments today and whose records will need to be refiled.

Exercise 2

Writing Activity

25 minutes

Answer the following questions regarding paper medical records and capabilities of EMR systems.

1. Which of the following would not be used to help prevent misfiling of medical records?
   a. Colored letter tabs for use with names
   b. Colored tabs for the last year seen in the office
   c. Outguides
   d. Alphabetic tabs in the filing system

2. The two paper filing systems most often used in a medical office are

   _____ and _____ filing.

3. Describe the differences in alphabetic and numeric filing systems.

4. Explain how color-coding enhances paper medical record systems?

5. List the five steps needed to prepare a paper medical record for filing.

    (1)

    (2)

    (3)

    (4)

    (5)

6. What steps can be followed for "finding" a misplaced paper medical record?

7. Explain the primary function of the following features of EMR software systems:

a. Specialty software

b. Appointment scheduler

c. Appointment reminder and confirmation

d. Prescription writer

e. Medical billing systems

f. Charge capture

g. Eligibility verification

h. Referral management

i. Laboratory order integration

j. Patient portal

LESSON 9

Insurance Forms and Verification

Reading Assignment: Chapter 18—Basics of Diagnostic Coding
Chapter 19—Basics of Procedural Coding
Chapter 20—Basics of Health Insurance
Chapter 21—The Health Insurance Claim Form

Patients: Shaunti Begay, Louise Parlet, John R. Simmons, Janet Jones, Jose Imero

Learning Objectives:

- Apply managed care policies and procedures to office billing and coding.
- Use third party guidelines for preparing insurance claims and collecting copayments.
- Verify insurance information and initiate a referral for a patient.
- Determine which diagnosis should be coded, and which should not, from patient documentation in the chart.
- Proofread an insurance claim form and identify errors that will affect claims processing.

Overview:

In this lesson you will perform the necessary steps to prepare a clean claim for insurance purposes and collecting copayments that are due to the practice. Completing these steps requires the correct use of managed care policies and procedures and the proper application of the office Policy Manual. A clean claim includes the appropriate diagnostic and procedural codes as well as the proper completion of the insurance claim form. You will proofread an insurance form and compare it with the information in the patient's chart and Encounter Form. You will indicate which boxes need corrections before the claim can be sent to the insurance company.

Exercise 1

Online Activity—Verifying Insurance for a New Patient

30 minutes

- Sign in to Mountain View Clinic.
- From the patient list, select **Shaunti Begay**.

- On the office map, highlight and click on **Reception**.

- At the Reception desk, click on **Policy** to open the office Policy Manual.

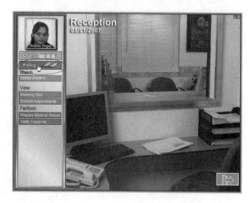

- Type "payment" in the search bar and click the magnifying glass once. This will take you to page 14 of the Policy Manual. Under the Telephone Policies heading, the sixth bullet reminds the medical assistant to inform patients that the copay or their portion of payment is due at the time of service.

- Type "patient insurance policies" in the search bar and click the magnifying glass once. This will take you to page 17 of the Policy Manual. Scroll up to adjust the page and read the policies that apply when patients have insurance coverage that is not accepted by the medical practice.

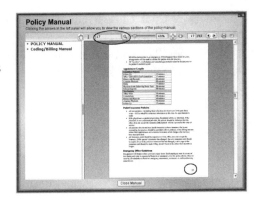

1. According to the Policy Manual, what information should be obtained from the patient when the appointment is made?

2. Why is it important for the medical assistant to verify whether the office is a preferred provider with the patient's insurance at the time the appointment is made?

- Scroll up to page 14 of the Policy Manual and read the section on Telephone Policies.

3. What does the Policy Manual state about collecting payments, copays, and percentages of charges for patient visits?

- Click **Close Manual** to return to the Reception desk.
- Click on **Patient Check-In** to view the video of Shaunti's arrival at the clinic.

- At the end of the video, click **Close** to return to the Reception desk.
- At the Reception desk, click on **Verify Insurance** to obtain the required information for Shaunti's visit.

- Select the appropriate question to ask Shaunti regarding her insurance; then click **Insurance Card(s)** to review the insurance cards on the next screen.

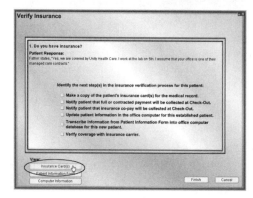

- Click **Finish** to return to the Reception desk.
- Click again on **Policy** to reopen the Policy Manual.
- From the menu on the left side of the screen, click on the arrow next to **Coding/Billing Manual**. The menu will expand. View the additional headings for that section of the Policy Manual.
- Click the arrow next to **Financial Policy** and select **Accepted Insurance Carriers** from the list. You may use the magnifying glass if needed.
- Click **Close Manual** to return to the Reception desk.

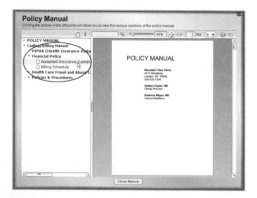

4. Was Kristin correct in stating that Mountain View Clinic was not a participating provider for Shaunti's insurance plan?

5. What did Shaunti's mother say about the information she gave the receptionist regarding their insurance coverage when she made the appointment?

6. What steps should the medical assistant have taken to avoid the confusion that occurred when Shaunti checked in?

→ • Click the exit arrow to leave the Reception desk.
  • From the Summary Menu, select **Return to Map**.

Exercise 2

Online Activity—Obtaining a Referral for an Established Patient

30 minutes

- Select **Louise Parlet** from the patient list. (*Note:* If you have exited the program, sign in again to Mountain View Clinic and select Louise Parlet from the patient list.)

- On the office map, highlight and click on **Check Out**.

- At the desk, click on **Patient Check-Out** to view the video.

- At the end of the video, click **Close** to return to the desk.

1. Why is it important that the medical assistant assist Ms. Parlet in obtaining approval from her insurance company for the referral to Dr. Lockett?

2. After receiving the precertification verification number, how should the medical assistant handle the verification number?

 • Next, click on **Charts** to open Ms. Parlet's medical record.
• Under the **Patient Medical Information** tab, select **3-Progress Notes** and read Dr. Hayler's notes regarding the examination.

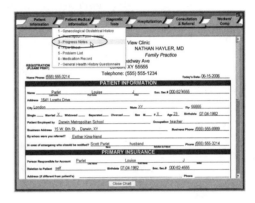

3. What instructions does Dr. Hayler give about the results of the lab work?

Critical Thinking Question

4. Do you think most insurance companies would reimburse a medical provider for a test if the test has already been completed at another facility?

 • Click **Close Chart** to return to the Check Out desk.
• Click the exit arrow; from the Summary Menu, select **Return to Map**.

Exercise 3

Online Activity—Choosing the Correct Diagnosis to Code for an Office Visit of a New Adult Patient

30 minutes

- Select **John R. Simmons** from the patient list. (*Note:* If you have exited the program, sign in again to Mountain View Clinic and select John R. Simmons from the patient list.)

- On the office map, highlight and click on **Billing and Coding**.

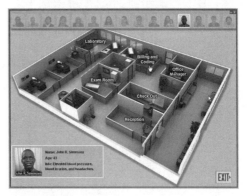

- At the Billing and Coding desk, click on **Encounter Form** to view the diagnostic and procedural information for Dr. Simmons' visit.

- Your instructor may ask you to use the ICD-10 to choose the correct numeric codes for the diagnoses listed.
- *Important:* Please remember that your codes will be from the ICD-10, not ICD-9, even though the Encounter Form says the clinic is using ICD-9.

1. In the ICD-9 section of the Encounter Form, which diagnoses are checked off for Dr. Simmons' visit?

2. Which of these diagnoses should receive an ICD-9 code? If there are any diagnoses that should not be coded, explain why not.

3. When should the Hemoccult test that the patient will collect at home be billed? Explain your answer.

 • Click **Finish** to close the Encounter Form and return to the Billing and Coding desk.

• Click on **Charts** to open Dr. Simmons' medical record.

• Under the **Patient Information** tab, select **5-Insurance Cards** from the drop-down menu.

4. What is meant by PCP?

5. What is meant by POS?

6. Using the information on the insurance cards found in the medical record, what is the copay on the patient's insurance? What is the payment rate on the secondary insurance?

7. Look at the back of both of the insurance cards. What do you notice when comparing the cards?

➡ • Click **Close Chart** to return to the Billing and Coding desk.
   • Click the exit arrow; from the Summary Menu, select **Return to Map**.

Exercise 4

Online Activity—Insurance Versus Workers' Compensation Claims

 30 minutes

- From the patient list, select **Janet Jones**. (*Note:* If you have exited the program, sign in again to Mountain View Clinic and select Janet Jones from the patient list.)

- On the office map, highlight and click on **Billing and Coding**.

- Click on **Charts** to open Janet Jones' medical record.
- Next, click on the **Patient Information** tab.

1. You will notice that in Ms. Jones' medical record, there is no information about private insurance coverage. Why is this important for this case?

2. If a patient says that he or she were injured at the workplace or has a work-related illness, what would the medical assistant need to do prior to escorting the patient to the examination room? Refer to the Workers' Compensation section in Chapter 20 of the textbook if you need help locating the answer.

 • Now click on the tab labeled **Workers' Comp**.

3. What information do you find under this tab in Ms. Jones' medical record?

4. Can you give an example of an injury or a problem for which the insurance company might not pay if the patient had previous problems with the same or a similar diagnosis?

Exercise 5

Other Activity—Proofreading and Critical Thinking Exercise

45 minutes

Jose Imero's insurance claim has been filled out by the medical assistant student. Your
responsibility is to review the insurance form and make sure it is correct prior to billing the
insurance company. There are several errors on the form. You will use the textbook, the Patient's
Information Form, the Insurance Card, the Progress Notes, and the Encounter Form to ensure
that everything on the form is correct. Review Chapter 21 in the textbook carefully before you
begin this exercise, and use it as a tool as you review the insurance form.

- From the patient list, select **Jose Imero**.
  (*Note:* If you have exited the program, sign in
  again to Mountain View Clinic and select Jose
  Imero from the patient list.)

- On the office map, highlight and click on **Billing
  and Coding**.

- Click on **Charts** to open Jose Imero's medical
  record. Then click on the **Patient Information**
  tab.
- From the drop-down menu, select **1-Patient
  Information Form** to review the patient's
  demographic information, which will be used to
  compare the first portion of the insurance form.
  When finished, select **2-Insurance Cards** to
  verify that the insurance identification numbers
  are correct.
- When you get to box 14 on the insurance claim
  form, click on the **Patient Medical Information**
  and choose **1-Progress Notes**. When finished,
  click **Close Chart**.

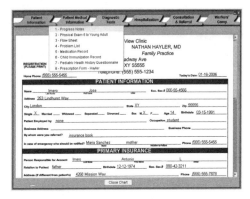

- When you get to box 24 on the insurance claim form, click on **Encounter Form** (under View) in the Billing and Coding office area to see what services the patient received. Click **Finish** when done.

- Select **Fee Schedule** (under View) in the Billing and Coding office area to make sure the insurance form has the correct amount for each service listed. Click **Finish** when done.

Important: The following instructions and notations will help as you go through the insurance form and make notations of errors.

It is indicated on Jose Imero's registration form that he is a student. For this exercise, consider his status as full-time student.

- Boxes 24 I and J should be left blank.
- For Box 25, you can locate the federal tax ID number on the Encounter Form at the top right-hand side.
- For Box 31, the office will file the claim the same date as the service was provided.
- For Box 33, the NPI number is 1234567899.

1. Below, list any errors you found as you reviewed Jose Imero's insurance claim form.

1500

HEALTH INSURANCE CLAIM FORM

APPROVED BY NATIONAL UNIFORM CLAIM COMMITTEE 08/05

CARRIER

☐☐☐ PICA   PICA ☐☐☐

1. MEDICARE ☐ MEDICAID ☐ TRICARE CHAMPUS ☐ CHAMPVA ☐ GROUP HEALTH PLAN ☒ FECA BLK LUNG ☐ OTHER ☐	1a. INSURED'S I.D. NUMBER (For Program in Item 1) **YAM 150221114**
2. PATIENT'S NAME (Last Name, First Name, Middle Initial) **Imero, Jose**	3. PATIENT'S BIRTH DATE **03 15 91** SEX M ☒ F ☐	4. INSURED'S NAME (Last Name, First Name, Middle Initial) **IMERO ANTONIO**
5. PATIENT'S ADDRESS (No., Street) **253 Lindhurst Way**	6. PATIENT RELATIONSHIP TO INSURED Self ☐ Spouse ☐ Child ☒ Other ☐	7. INSURED'S ADDRESS (No., Street) **4628 Mission Way**
CITY **London** STATE **XY**	8. PATIENT STATUS Single ☐ Married ☐ Other ☐	CITY **Trumball** STATE **YZ**
ZIP CODE **55555** TELEPHONE **(555) 555-5455**	Employed ☐ Full-Time Student ☒ Part-Time Student ☐	ZIP CODE **99999** TELEPHONE **(555) 555-7878**
9. OTHER INSURED'S NAME	10. IS PATIENT'S CONDITION RELATED TO:	11. INSURED'S POLICY GROUP OR FECA NUMBER **1822**
a. OTHER INSURED'S POLICY OR GROUP NUMBER	a. EMPLOYMENT? YES ☐ NO ☒	a. INSURED'S DATE OF BIRTH **12 12 74** SEX M ☒ F ☐
b. OTHER INSURED'S DATE OF BIRTH SEX M ☐ F ☐	b. AUTO ACCIDENT? YES ☐ NO ☒ PLACE (State)	b. EMPLOYER'S NAME OR SCHOOL NAME **Sunshine Foods**
c. EMPLOYER'S NAME OR SCHOOL NAME	c. OTHER ACCIDENT? YES ☒ NO ☐	c. INSURANCE PLAN NAME OR PROGRAM NAME **Blue Cross/Blue Shield**
d. INSURANCE PLAN NAME OR PROGRAM NAME	10d. RESERVED FOR LOCAL USE	d. IS THERE ANOTHER HEALTH BENEFIT PLAN? YES ☐ NO ☒

READ BACK OF FORM BEFORE COMPLETING & SIGNING THIS FORM.

12. PATIENT'S OR AUTHORIZED PERSON'S SIGNATURE
SIGNED **Signature on File**   DATE

13. INSURED'S OR AUTHORIZED PERSON'S SIGNATURE
SIGNED **Signature on File**

14. DATE OF CURRENT ILLNESS/INJURY/PREGNANCY **05 01 07**	15. IF PATIENT HAS HAD SAME OR SIMILAR ILLNESS	16. DATES PATIENT UNABLE TO WORK FROM TO
17. NAME OF REFERRING PROVIDER 17a. 17b. NPI		18. HOSPITALIZATION DATES FROM TO
19. RESERVED FOR LOCAL USE		20. OUTSIDE LAB? YES ☐ NO ☒ $ CHARGES
21. DIAGNOSIS OR NATURE OF ILLNESS OR INJURY 1. Open Wound L foot 8 cm w/ complications 3. 2. 4.		22. MEDICAID RESUBMISSION CODE ORIGINAL REF. NO. 23. PRIOR AUTHORIZATION NUMBER

24. A. DATE(S) OF SERVICE From / To	B. PLACE OF SERVICE	C. EMG	D. PROCEDURES, SERVICES, OR SUPPLIES CPT/HCPCS / MODIFIER	E. DIAGNOSIS POINTER	F. $ CHARGES	G. DAYS OR UNITS	H. EPSDT	I. ID QUAL	J. RENDERING PROVIDER ID. #
1 05 05 07 / 05 01 07	11		Est. visit, Level II	laceration	45 00	1	N	NPI	
2			Tetanus	laceration	15 00	1	N	NPI	
3			Immun. Single	laceration	25 00	1	N	NPI	
4			Surgical Tray	laceration	15 00	1	N	NPI	
5			Wound Repair	laceration	175 00	1	N	NPI	
6								NPI	

25. FEDERAL TAX I.D. NUMBER **123456789** SSN ☐ EIN ☒	26. PATIENT'S ACCOUNT NO.	27. ACCEPT ASSIGNMENT? YES ☒ NO ☐	28. TOTAL CHARGE $ 275 00	29. AMOUNT PAID $ 25 00	30. BALANCE DUE $ 250 00

31. SIGNATURE OF PHYSICIAN OR SUPPLIER **SOF** SIGNED DATE 05012007	32. SERVICE FACILITY LOCATION INFORMATION **44 BROADWAY LONDON, XY, 55555** a. NPI b.	33. BILLING PROVIDER INFO & PH # ( ) **NATHAN HAYLER MD 4412 BROADWAY LONDON, XY, 55555** a. 1234567899 b.

NUCC Instruction Manual available at: www.nucc.org   APPROVED OMB-0938-0999 FORM CMS-1500 (08/05)

Bookkeeping

Reading Assignment: Chapter 22—Professional Fees, Billing, and Collecting
- How Fees Are Determined
- Bookkeeping Computations Used on Patient Accounts
- Comparison of Manual and Computerized Bookkeeping Systems
- Special Bookkeeping Entries
- Payment Options
- Collection Techniques
- Using Outside Collection Assistance

Chapter 23—Banking Services and Procedures

Chapter 24—Financial and Practice Management
- What Is Accounting?

Patients: All

Learning Objectives:

- Post daily entries on the day sheet and prepare bank deposits at the end of the day.
- Process credit balances, NSF checks, and checks from collection agencies.
- Process credit balances and complete the necessary steps to process a refund, including preparation of a check.
- Reconcile a bank statement.
- Maintain a petty cash fund.
- Discuss the maintenance of records for accounting and banking purposes.
- Discuss the importance of managing accounts payable promptly.

Overview:

In this lesson the basic bookkeeping procedures will be accomplished. All patients will be added to the day sheet, along with the payments and the NSF checks received in today's mail. A deposit record will be prepared. The steps for the reconciliation of the bank statement and maintenance of records for accounting purposes will also be covered.

Exercise 1

Online Activity—Posting Charges to Ledger Cards

 30 minutes

- Sign in to Mountain View Clinic.
- Select **Jade Wong** from the patient list.

- On the office map, highlight and click on **Billing and Coding**.

- In the Billing and Coding office, select **Encounter Form** to review the services that will be billed for Jade's visit.

1. a. Using the Encounter Form for Jade Wong, begin completing the blank ledger card below.
   b. In the column marked Professional Service, list each individual service provided, but do not enter any fee or balance information.
   c. After the last service has been entered, be sure to record that the copay was collected and enter the amount in the Payment column.

Patient Name:
Insurance Type:

Date	Professional Service	Fee ($)	Payment ($)	Adj. ($)	Prev. Bal. ($)	New Balance ($)
Totals						

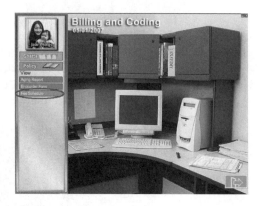

- • Click **Finish** to return to Billing and Coding.
- • Now click on **Fee Schedule** to review the amount Mountain View Clinic charges for various services and procedures.

- • Again using the ledger card on the previous page, fill in the fees charged for the listed services and calculate the balances.

Important: The balance should be corrected line by line as each service or payment is added or subtracted.

2. After filling in the services, fees, and payments for Jade's current visit, should the ledger card be totaled as indicated at the bottom of the card? Refer to the textbook, if needed, and explain your answer.

3. How did the medical assistant know what Jade's copay was?

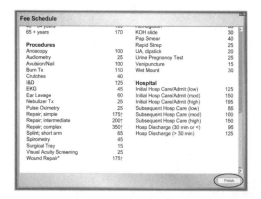

- • Click **Finish** to close the Fee Schedule; then click the exit arrow to leave Billing and Coding.

- • On the Summary Menu, click on **Return to Map** and continue to the next exercise.

Exercise 2

Online Activity—Posting Entries to a Day Sheet

 60 minutes

1. In this activity you will post charges and payments for the patients who were seen in the office today, using the day sheet on the next page. Note that the distribution columns are used to indicate which physician, Dr. Hayler or Dr. Meyer, provided care to the patient. The amount of money the patient paid should be written in one of those columns in addition to the payment column.

   a. In the Patient Name column on the blank day sheet on the next page, list the patients in the following order: Jade Wong, Louise Parlet, Hu Huang, Rhea Davison, Jesus Santo, Jean Deere, Tristan Tsosie, Wilson Metcalf, Renee Anderson, Jose Imero, Shaunti Begay, Janet Jones, Kevin McKinzie, John R. Simmons, and Teresa Hernandez.

   b. Select Jade Wong from the patient list. Then click on **Check Out** on the office map. Once in the Check Out area, open the **Encounter Form**.

   c. Using one line per patient, complete each column on the day sheet using the Total Charges, Previous Balance, and Amount Received information listed on the Encounter Form. Refer back to the ledger card in Exercise 1 to confirm your totals. (*Note:* Unlike the ledger card, the Professional Service column on the day sheet is a summary description of the visit.)

   d. For the purposes of this exercise, also make a note next to each patient's name to indicate whether the patient paid by cash, check, or credit card. If payment was made by check, include the check number.

   e. Repeat the above steps by selecting each patient listed on the day sheet and opening his or her Encounter Form at Check Out. As you finish each patient's portion of the day sheet, click **Finish** to close the Encounter Form. Click the exit arrow to leave Check Out and **Return to Map** to select the next patient.

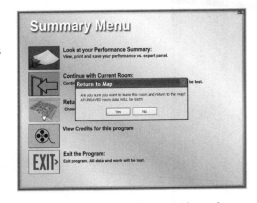

   f. When you finish recording the information for the last patient on the list, remain at the office map to continue with the next question.

Mountain View Clinic
Daysheet

Distribution		Patient's Name	Old Balance	New Balance	Adjustment	Payment	Fee	Professional Service	Date
Dr. Meyer	Dr. Hayler								

TOTALS

TOTALS

- From the office map, click on **Reception**. (The selected patient should be Teresa Hernandez, the last patient on the list in question 1.)
- At the Reception desk, click on **Incoming Mail** to view the day's correspondence.

2. a. View each piece of incoming mail; then on the blank day sheet on the next page, record any payments received by the clinic and any charges paid by the clinic in the appropriate columns.

b. Be sure to include a description of the payment/charge and the patient's name.

c. For the purposes of this exercise, make a note of the bank and check number next to the name of any patient who paid by check.

d. To complete the remaining columns, first click **Finish** to close the mail.

e. Next, click the exit arrow and **Return to Map**.

f. Click on **Office Manager** and then on **Day Sheet** (under View) to find any previous balance information for the patients whose accounts were updated from the mail received.

g. Mark Bonsel's previous account balance was zero ("0") before you received the NSF check. The NSF check shows that it was paid on April 7, 2007, but it does not indicate what it was for, other than a balance. Assume it was for a level II new patient visit, which would be $65.00 on the date of April 7, 2007.

Note: A copy of Sarah Anita's EOB from Blue Cross/Blue Shield was received in the mail. The insurance payment and adjustment were already posted on the day sheet and on her ledger in the office manager's section of the Office. The copy of the EOB in the mail will not need to be posted again.

Recalculate the balance and record it in the New Balance column.

Mountain View Clinic
Daysheet

Date	Professional Service	Fee	Payment	Adjustment	New Balance	Old Balance	Patient's Name	Distribution	
								Dr. Hayler	Dr. Meyer

TOTALS

TOTALS

• Click **Finish** and continue to the next exercise.

Exercise 3

 Writing Activity—Preparing a Bank Deposit

15 minutes

Using the information recorded in the completed day sheets in Exercise 2, you will now prepare a bank deposit (both front and back) for the accounts receivable for the day. Be sure the total on the deposit slip balances with the total of receivables on the day sheet.

1. Below, complete the front side of the deposit slip.

DEPOSIT SLIP

Clarion National Bank
90 Grape Vine Road
London, XY 55555-0001

Mountain View Clinic
4412 Broadway
London, XY 55555

Date: _____

CASH			TOTAL
	Currency	$_____	
	Coin	$_____	$_____
	Total Cash		$_____
CHECKS	See other side for detail		$_____
- CASH REC'D			$_____
NET DEPOSIT			$_____

SIGN HERE IN TELLER'S PRESENCE FOR CASH RECEIVED

2. Below, complete the back portion of the bank deposit slip. (*Note:* The bank number cannot be obtained from the day sheet. For the purposes of this exercise, use the check number as a substitute.)

BANK DEPOSIT DETAIL

PAYMENTS

BANK NUMBER	BY CHECK OR PMO		BY COIN OR CURRENCY		CREDIT CARD	
TOTALS						
CURRENCY						
COIN						
CHECKS						
CREDIT CARDS						
TOTAL RECEIPTS						
LESS CREDIT CARD $						
TOTAL DEPOSIT						
DEPOSIT DATE						

Exercise 4

Online Activity—Processing a Credit Balance

20 minutes

- Remain in the manager's office and click on **Day Sheet**. (*Note:* If you have exited the manager's office and are at the office map, click on **Office Manager** and then click on **Day Sheet**.)

1. Two patients listed on the day sheet have overpaid, which resulted in a credit balance denoted by a parenthesis around the amount that was overpaid. Betsy Dunworthy overpaid by $20.00, and her refund was already processed. What is the name of the other patient who should receive a refund, and how much money should he receive?

2. Using the blank check below, process the outstanding refund for payment.

173975				
		MOUNTAIN VIEW CLINIC		173975
		4412 Broadway		94-721/224
DATE:		London, XY 55555	Date:	
TO:				
FOR:		Pay to the order of:		
ACCOUNT NO.				
AMOUNT PAID	$		Dollars $	
		Clarion National Bank		
		Member FDIC		
		90 Grape Vine Road		Authorized Signature
		London, XY 55555-0001		

||" 005503 ||" 446782011 ||" 678800470

- Click **Finish** to return to the manager's office.

Exercise 5

Online Activity—Maintaining Petty Cash Fund

30 minutes

- In the office manager's office, click on **Petty Cash Log**. (*Note:* If you have exited the office manager's office and are at the office map, click on **Office Manager** and select **Petty Cash Log**.)

1. Petty cash was used to pay for the mailing of a certified letter. What are the receipt number and date from this transaction?

2. On 5-1-07, the administrative medical assistant was asked to obtain soft drinks for an office celebration to be held that afternoon. These were bought at Sav-A-Grocery for the amount of $24.56. She also mailed a large package at the post office. The cost for mailing the package was $15.08. Using the form below, fill out the first petty cash voucher.

Date: _____   No.: __109__

PETTY CASH VOUCHER

For: _____

Charge to: _____

_____

Approved by: Received by:

_____   _____
Authorized Signature

3. Now fill out the second petty cash voucher.

Date: _____   No.: **110**

PETTY CASH VOUCHER

For: _____

Charge to: _____

_____

Approved by: Received by:

_____   _____
Authorized Signature

4. Using the completed petty cash vouchers from questions 2 and 3, update the petty cash log below accordingly. Be sure to distribute the expenses to the proper expense column.

NO.	DATE	DESCRIPTION	AMOUNT	OFFICE EXP.	AUTO.	MISC.	BALANCE
	2/16/2007	Fund Established (check #217)					200.00
101	2/24/2007	Certified Letter	3.74	3.74			196.26
102	3/1/2007	Staff Meeting/Lunch	24.60			24.60	171.66
103	3/6/2007	Coffee	4.32			4.32	167.34
104	3/8/2007	Tympanic Thermometer	38.00	38.00			129.34
105	3/8/2007	Parking Fee	6.00		6.00		123.34
106	4/1/2007	Staff Meeting/Lunch	27.43			27.43	95.91
107	4/13/2007	Miscellaneous Supplies	9.01	9.01			86.90
108	4/21/2007	Patient Birthday Cards	12.17	12.17			74.73

5. Office policy states that petty cash should be replenished when the amount falls below $50. Use the blank check below to replenish the petty cash fund to the full $200 balance as required by office policy. Then, using the updated petty cash log in question 4, verify the petty cash fund balances by totaling all the columns, and add this transaction to the log.

173976

DATE:	
TO:	
FOR:	
ACCOUNT NO.	
AMOUNT PAID	$

MOUNTAIN VIEW CLINIC
4412 Broadway
London, XY 55555

173976

94-724224

Date: _____

Pay to the order of: _____

_____ Dollars $ _____

Clarion National Bank
Member FDIC
90 Grape Vine Road
London, XY 55555-0001

Authorized Signature

||⬛ 005503 ||⬛ ⑂678201 ||⬛ 678800⑂70

- Click **Finish** to return to the manager's office.
- Click the exit arrow; from the Summary Menu, select **Return to Map**.
- On the office map, select **Jose Imero** from the patient list and click on **Check Out**.

- At the Check Out desk, select **Patient Check Out** (under Watch) to view the video.

6. What are the ethical implications of Kristin asking another medical assistant for money from petty cash?

 • Click **Close** to return to the Check Out desk.
• Click the exit arrow; from the Summary Menu, select **Return to Map**.

Exercise 6

 Online Activity—Managing Accounts Payable

 30 minutes

• Using any patient from the patient list, click on **Reception** on the office map.
• Select **Incoming Mail** (under View) and review pieces 8 and 9.

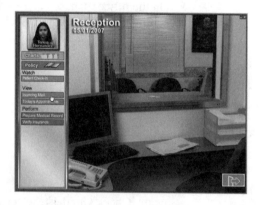

1. Indicate whether each of the following statements is true or false.

   a. _____ When accounts payable arrive, the date for payment with discounts should be noted.

   b. _____ It really does not matter what day of the month an accounts payable payment is made, as long as it is paid before the next billing cycle.

   c. _____ Invoices should be marked with the date and check number, as well as the initials of the person preparing the check.

   d. _____ All accounts payables should be checked against invoices and packing slips before payment is made to ensure that everything ordered was received.

   e. _____ All vendors will present invoices before payment is due.

2. Which of the following information does the accounts payable person need to correctly process and post the payment of the invoices (pieces 8 and 9 of the incoming mail)? Select all that apply.

_____ Invoice number

_____ Company name

_____ Name of the customer service representative

_____ Date of the check

_____ Account number

_____ Company address

_____ Company phone number

_____ Name of the company's bank

_____ Company's bank account number

_____ Type of expense

_____ Amount of the check

_____ Invoice date

_____ Check number

➤ • Click **Finish** to close the mail and return to the Reception desk.
  • Click the exit arrow; from the Summary Menu, select **Return to Map**.

Exercise 7

Online Activity—Reconciling a Bank Statement

30 minutes

The clinic's bank statement arrives in today's mail. This is found in the manager's office. She is extremely busy and asks that you take the time to reconcile the statement for her.

- On the office map, click on **Office Manager** to enter the manager's office. (*Note:* For this task, it does not matter which patient is selected. You may continue with Jose Imero from the previous exercise.)
- From the menu on the left, select **Bank Statement**.

1. a. Using the check ledger below, review the bank statement and check off each deposit, check, withdrawal, ATM transaction, or credit listed on the statement.

   b. If the statement shows any interest paid to the account, service charges, bank fees, automatic payments, or ATM transactions withdrawn from the account that are not listed on the check ledger, make an entry for those items now and recalculate the account balance in the ledger.

No.	Date	Description	Payment/ Debit	Ref	Deposit/ Credit	Balance
1216	4/5/2007	Rocke Medical	$625.00			$9,264.35
1217	4/5/2007	Wal Store	$38.46			$9,225.89
1218	4/6/2007	Lorenz Equipment	$1006.00			$8,219.89
1219	4/8/2007	Office Station	$199.43			$8,020.46
	4/10/2007	Dep. Daily Trans			$1,050.00	$10,833.46
1220	4/10/2007	West Electric	$93.99			$7,926.47
	4/12/2007	Dep. Daily Trans			$2,008.00	$9,934.47
1221	4/12/2007	Office Depot	$102.01			$9,832.46
1222	4/12/2007	Video Inc.	$49.00			$9,783.46
	4/15/2007	Dep. Daily Trans			$1,002.00	$11,835.46
1223	4/17/2007	Bonus	$200.00			$12,560.46
1224	4/17/2007	Bonus	$200.00			$12,360.46
1225	4/17/2007	Bonus	$200.00			$12,160.46
	4/20/2007	Dep. Daily Trans			$925.00	$12,760.46
1226	4/21/2007	Jamison Medical	$2,024.00			$10,136.26
1227	4/22/2007	Healthy Living Magazine	$32.95			$10,103.31
1228	4/22/2007	Greater London Electric	$422.00			$9,681.31
1229	4/24/2007	Office Station	$344.70			$9,336.61
1230	4/25/2007	Summer Oxygen	$230.99			$9,105.62
	4/27/2007	Dep. Daily Trans			$1,550.00	$10,655.62

2. Now complete the bank reconciliation worksheet below.

THIS WORKSHEET IS PROVIDED TO HELP YOU BALANCE YOUR ACCOUNT

1. Go through your register and mark each check, withdrawal, Express ATM transaction, payment, deposit or other credit listed on your statement. Be sure that your register shows any interest paid into your account, and any service charges, bank fees, automatic payments, or Express Transfers withdrawn from your account during this statement period.

2. Using the chart below, list any outstanding checks, Express ATM withdrawals, payments or any other withdrawals (including any from previous months) that are listed in your register but are not shown on this statement.

3. Balance your account by filling in the spaces below.

ITEMS OUTSTANDING		
NUMBER	**AMOUNT**	
TOTAL		

ENTER

The ENDING BALANCE shown on this statement -------------------------------- $ _____ __

ADD

Any deposits listed in your register or $ _____ __
transfers into your account which are $ _____ __
not shown on this statement $ _____ __
                                            +$ _____ __

TOTAL-----------------------------------+ $ _____ __

CALCULATE THE SUBTOTAL --- $ _____ __

SUBTRACT

The total outstanding checks and
Withdrawals from the chart at the left --- $ _____ __

CALCULATE THE ENDING BALANCE

This amount should be the same as
The current balance shown in your
Check register --- $ _____ __

Payroll Procedures

/OO **Reading Assignment:** Chapter 24—Financial and Practice Management
- Payroll Records

Patients: None

Learning Objectives:

- Process the employee payroll.
- Locate federal tax withholding resources by using the Internet

Overview:

For administrative medical assistants, the task of preparing an employee payroll may be a routine function. This lesson will give you practice in preparing a payroll for employees.

Exercise 1

Online Activity—Processing Payroll

20 minutes

- Sign in to Mountain View Clinic.
- On the office map, highlight and click on **Office Manager** to enter the manager's office. (*Note:* You do not need to select a patient for this exercise.)

- Click on **Payroll Forms** to view the office payroll records.

- The time sheet for employee Cathy Wright will appear first. Review and confirm that the number of hours has been calculated correctly.
- Next, click on the down arrow next to Person and select **Susan Bronski**.
- Review Susan Bronski's time sheet and confirm the calculations for the number of hours she worked.

1. Cathy Wright's total number of hours worked: _____

   Susan Bronski's total number of hours worked: _____

2. Cathy Wright has been employed by the clinic for 10 years. Her salary is $18.00 per hour for the first 80 hours and $27.00 per hour for any hours over 80 during the 2-week pay period. Compute the gross pay for Cathy for the 2-week period.

3. Susan Bronski is a relatively new employee who is making $15.00 per hour for the first 80 hours and $20 per hour for hours over 80. Compute the gross pay for Susan for the 2-week period.

• Now review the W-4 form filled out by each employee.
• To view Cathy Wright's W-4 form, first make sure her name is selected from the drop-down menu next to Person. Next, click on the down arrow next to Form and select **W-4**. Review her form.
• To view Susan Bronski's W-4 form, select her name from the drop-down menu next to Person.

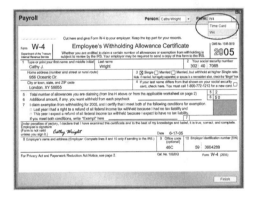

4. Cathy Wright elected to have her federal taxes withheld under which designation?

_____ Single

_____ Married

_____ Married, but withhold at the higher single rate

5. The number of allowances claimed by Cathy Wright is _____.

6. Did Cathy Wright elect to have any additional money withheld from her paycheck for federal taxes? If yes, how much?

7. Susan Bronski will have her federal taxes withheld under which designation?

_____ Single

_____ Married

_____ Married, but withhold at the higher single rate

8. The number of allowances claimed by Susan Bronski is _____.

9. Did Susan Bronski elect to have any additional money withheld from her paycheck for federal taxes? If yes, how much?

Exercise 2

Writing Activity—Calculating Net Pay

30 minutes

The IRS updates the federal tax tables each year. The tables we are using for this activity are 2010 tables for Single and Married Persons Biweekly Payroll (you will choose which table to use based on the employees filing status). Go to the Evolve course website. Click on Course Documents to view the 2010 tax tables. If you are instructed by your teacher to obtain the most recent copy of the schedules, go to the IRS website at www.irs.gov. Each state may have its own amount for the state withholding, but for this exercise we will use 1%.

1. Calculate the federal withholding allowance for Cathy Wright and Susan Bronski.

   Total withholding allowance (federal) for Cathy Wright: _____

   Total withholding allowance (federal) for Susan Bronski: _____

2. Now subtract the total withholding allowance from each employee's gross pay to calculate the adjusted gross pay.

   Cathy Wright's adjusted gross pay: _____

   Susan Bronski's adjusted gross pay: _____

3. Account for the following additional deductions for Cathy Wright: Medicare = 1.45%, Social Security = 6.2%, Health Insurance = $125 per pay, State Income Tax = 1%, Retirement Plan = $150 per pay.

Federal Income Tax	
Medicare	
Social Security	
Health Insurance	
State Income Tax	
Retirement Savings Plan	

4. What is the net pay for Cathy Wright? _____

5. a. Using the correct tax table, calculate the correct deductions for Susan Bronski, who will file as head of household.

b. Account for the following additional deductions for Susan Bronski: Medicare = 1.45%, Social Security = 6.2%, Health Insurance = $175 per pay, State Income Tax = 1%, Savings Plan = $50 per pay period, Additional Tax Withholding from W-4 = $190.00.

Federal Income Tax	
Medicare	
Social Security	
Health Insurance	
State Income Tax	
Retirement Savings Plan	
Additional Tax Withholding	

6. What is the net pay for Susan Bronski? _____

Exercise 3

Online Activity—Writing the Check for Payroll

15 minutes

You are now ready to prepare and issue the payroll checks for Cathy Wright and Susan Bronski. To obtain the correct ending date for the pay period, return to the employees' time sheets by clicking on **Payroll Forms** in the manager's office. Date the checks for the Monday following the end of the pay period.

1. Prepare Cathy Wright's payroll check below.

PERIOD ENDING	EARNINGS			DEDUCTIONS										NET PAY
HOURS WORKED REG. OT	REGULAR	OVERTIME	TOTAL	FEDERAL INCOME TAX	FICA TAX	STATE INCOME TAX	SDI TAX	HEALTH INS.	SAVINGS	MEDICARE	MISC DED.	TOTAL DED.	AMOUNT	

CHECK # 173977   **Employee:**

MOUNTAIN VIEW CLINIC   173977
4412 Broadway
London, XY 55555   94-72/1224

Date: _____

Pay to the order of: _____

_____ *Dollars* | $ _____ |

Clarion National Bank
Member FDIC
90 Grape Vine Road
London, XY 55555-0001   *Authorized Signature*

⑅ 005503 ⑅ 4⑅678⑅2011 ⑅ 678800470

2. Prepare Susan Bronski's payroll check below.

PERIOD ENDING	EARNINGS			DEDUCTIONS								NET PAY	
HOURS WORKED REG. OT	REGULAR	OVERTIME	TOTAL	FEDERAL INCOME TAX	FICA TAX	STATE INCOME TAX	SDI TAX	HEALTH INS.	SAVINGS	MEDICARE	MISC DED.	TOTAL DED.	AMOUNT

CHECK # 173978   Employee:

MOUNTAIN VIEW CLINIC   173978
4412 Broadway
London, XY 55555   94-72/1224

                                                          Date: _____

Pay to the order of: _____

_____ Dollars $ [   ]

Clarion National Bank
        Member FDIC
90 Grape Vine Road   _____
London, XY 55555-0001   Authorized Signature

      ||⸱ 005503 ||⸱ 446782011 ||⸱ 678800470